ATKINS DIET COOKBOOK 2024

1800-DAYS OF EASY, TASTY RECIPES FOR WEIGHT LOSS AND HEALTHY LIVING

DR. LESLIE J. STEEN

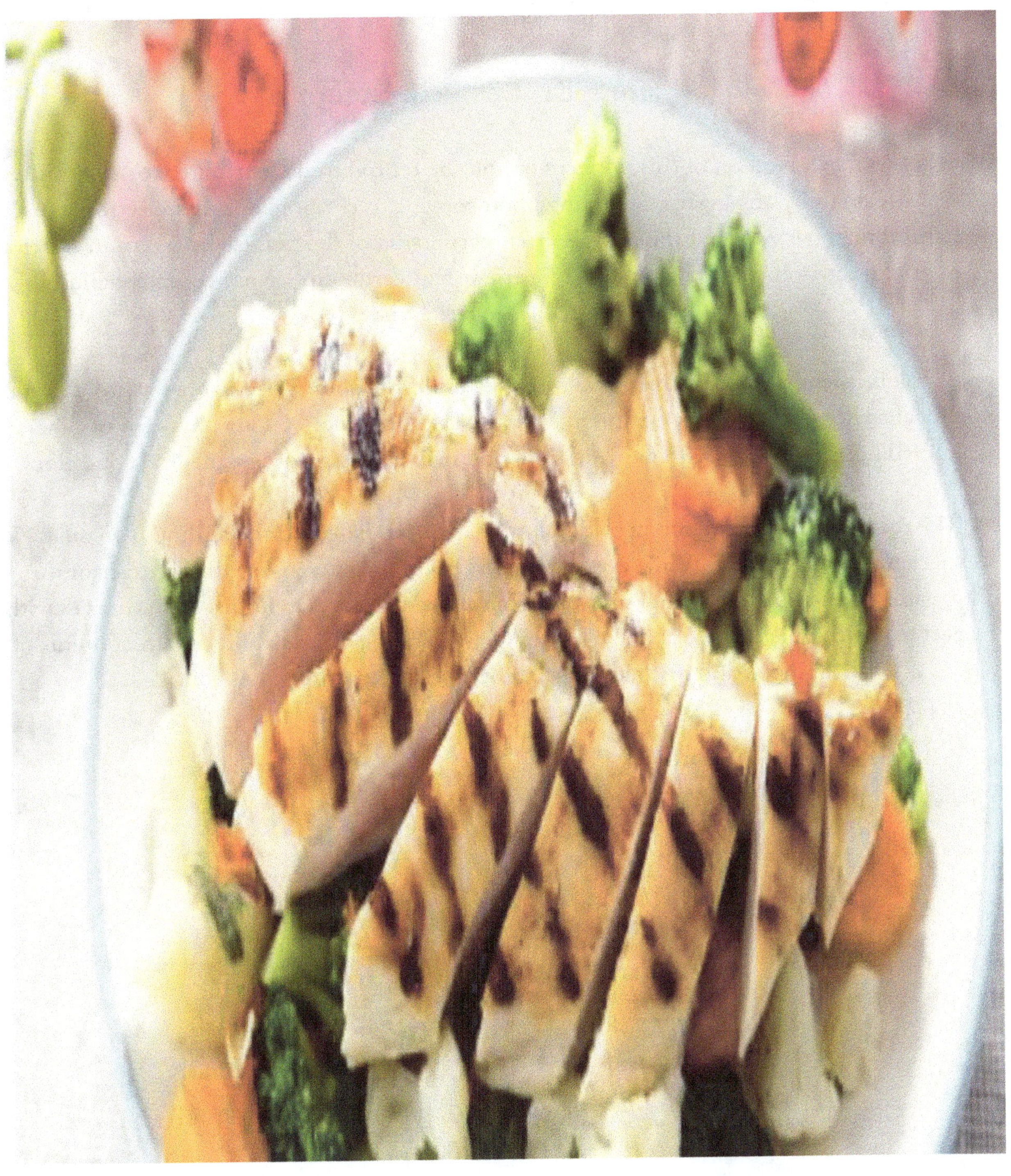

2

DR. LESLIE J. STEEN

COPYRIGHT

© 2024 by **Dr. Leslie J. Steen**

ABOUT THE AUTHOR

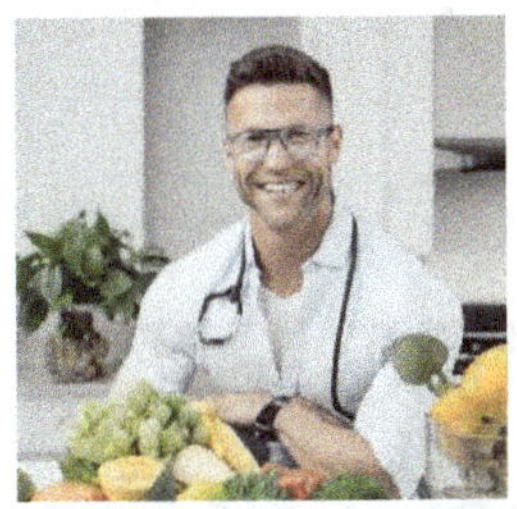

Dr. Leslie J. Steen is a passionate and dedicated dietitian with extensive experience in the field of nutrition and wellness. With a deep-rooted commitment to helping others achieve their health goals, Dr. Steen has dedicated his career to empowering individuals to make informed choices about their diet and lifestyle.

Dr. Steen holds a Doctorate in Dietetics and has spent over 2 decades working in various clinical and community settings, helping individuals of all ages and backgrounds improve their health through nutrition. His expertise encompasses a wide range of areas, including weight management, chronic disease prevention and management, sports nutrition, and nutritional counseling.

Throughout his career, Dr. Steen has been a vocal advocate for evidence-based nutrition education and has contributed to numerous research studies and publications in the field. He is deeply committed to staying abreast of the latest developments and research in nutrition science to ensure that his clients receive the most up-to-date and effective guidance.

In addition to his clinical work, Dr. Steen is also a sought-after speaker and educator, regularly delivering seminars, workshops, and presentations on topics related to nutrition, health, and wellness. He is known for his engaging and informative teaching style, which empowers audiences to take charge of their health and make positive changes in their lives.

As the author of the "Atkins Diet Cookbook 2024," Dr. Steen brings together his expertise in nutrition and passion for delicious, wholesome food to provide readers with a comprehensive guide to following the Atkins diet. Through this cookbook, he aims to inspire and empower individuals to embrace a low-carb lifestyle while enjoying flavorful and satisfying meals.

TABLE OF CONTENTS

INTRODUCTION

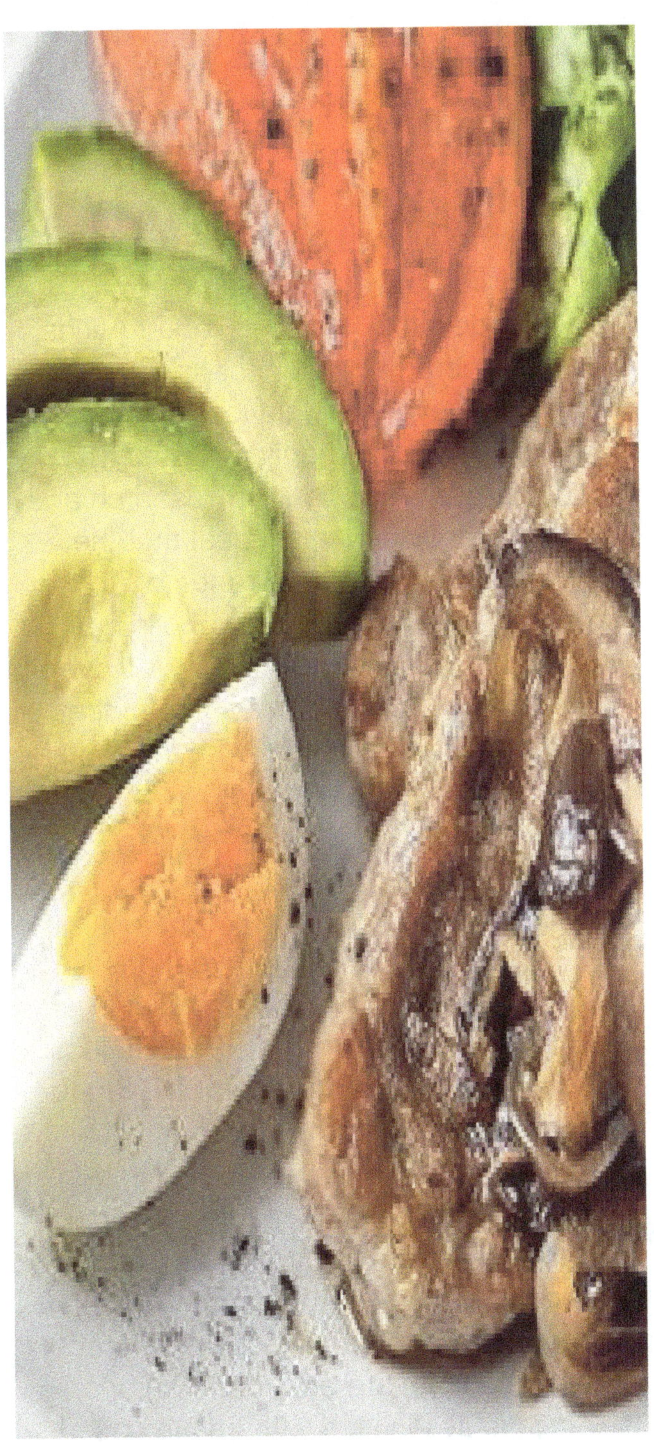

ABOUT THE ATKINS DIET

The Atkins Diet, developed by Dr. Robert Atkins in the early 1970s, is a low-carbohydrate eating plan designed to promote weight loss and improve overall health. Over the years, it has gained widespread popularity and has evolved into various iterations, each with its own focus and guidelines. The fundamental principle of the Atkins Diet remains reducing carbohydrate intake while emphasizing protein and healthy fats.

ORIGINS AND EVOLUTION

Dr. Robert Atkins, an American cardiologist, introduced the Atkins Diet through his book "Dr. Atkins' Diet Revolution" in 1972. His approach challenged conventional dietary wisdom by advocating for a low-carbohydrate, high-fat diet as a means of weight loss and improving metabolic health.

Initially met with skepticism from mainstream medical and nutritional communities, the Atkins Diet gained momentum as individuals reported significant weight loss and improvements in various health markers. Subsequent editions of Dr. Atkins' books, along with scientific research supporting the efficacy of low-carbohydrate diets, contributed to its growing acceptance.

PRINCIPLES OF THE ATKINS DIET

The Atkins Diet is based on the premise that reducing carbohydrate intake forces the body to burn stored fat for fuel, leading to weight loss. The diet consists of four phases:

1. Induction Phase: This initial phase restricts carbohydrate intake to 20-25 grams per day, primarily from non-starchy vegetables. Dieters consume ample protein, fats, and low-carb vegetables to jump-start ketosis, a metabolic state where the body burns fat for energy.

2. Balancing Phase: In this phase, carbohydrate intake is gradually increased as long as weight loss continues steadily. Individuals experiment to determine their personal carbohydrate tolerance level while maintaining weight loss progress.

3. Pre-Maintenance Phase: Carbohydrate intake is further increased to fine-tune weight loss and transition to a sustainable long-term eating pattern. This phase prepares individuals for the maintenance phase by introducing more variety into their diet.

4. Maintenance Phase: Once weight loss goals are achieved, individuals maintain their desired weight by adhering to a sustainable low-carbohydrate lifestyle. This phase emphasizes balance, variety, and flexibility in food choices while prioritizing whole, nutrient-dense foods

BENEFITS OF THE ATKINS DIET

The Atkins Diet, a low-carbohydrate eating plan developed by Dr. Robert Atkins, has garnered attention for its potential benefits beyond weight loss. While initially known primarily for its efficacy in shedding excess pounds, research and anecdotal evidence suggest that the Atkins Diet may offer a range of advantages related to metabolic health, energy levels, mental clarity, and overall well-being. Let's explore some of the key benefits associated with this dietary approach:

1. Weight Loss and Weight Management:

One of the primary reasons individuals turn to the Atkins Diet is its effectiveness in promoting weight loss. By significantly reducing carbohydrate intake and prioritizing protein and healthy fats, the body is forced to burn stored fat for energy, leading to rapid and sustainable weight loss for many people. Moreover, the Atkins Diet has been shown to target visceral fat, the dangerous fat stored around organs, which is associated with an increased risk of metabolic disorders and cardiovascular disease.

Beyond initial weight loss, the Atkins Diet offers a structured approach to weight management. Through its phased approach, individuals learn to identify their carbohydrate tolerance levels, make informed food choices, and maintain their desired weight over the long term.

2. Improved Metabolic Health:

Low-carbohydrate diets like Atkins have been linked to improvements in various markers of metabolic health. By reducing carbohydrate intake and moderating insulin levels, the Atkins Diet can enhance insulin sensitivity, helping the body better regulate blood sugar levels and reducing the risk of insulin resistance and type 2 diabetes. Additionally, studies have shown that low-carbohydrate diets may lead to favorable changes in blood lipid profiles, including increased HDL (good) cholesterol levels and decreased triglycerides, which are associated with a lower risk of cardiovascular disease.

3. Steady Energy Levels:

Unlike high-carbohydrate diets that can lead to fluctuations in blood sugar levels and energy crashes, the Atkins Diet provides a steady source of energy throughout the day. By prioritizing protein and healthy fats, which are digested more slowly than carbohydrates, the Atkins Diet helps maintain stable blood sugar levels and sustained energy levels. This can result in improved focus, mental clarity, and productivity, without the highs and lows associated with sugar and carbohydrate consumption.

4. Enhanced Satiety and Appetite Control:

Protein and healthy fats, the cornerstone of the Atkins Diet, are known for their satiating properties. By including ample amounts of protein-rich foods such as meat, fish, eggs, and dairy, along with healthy fats from sources like avocados, nuts, seeds, and olive oil, the Atkins Diet helps individuals feel fuller for longer periods and reduces cravings for unhealthy, high-carbohydrate snacks. This increased satiety can lead to naturally lower calorie intake, making it easier to adhere to a reduced-calorie diet without feeling deprived.

5. Reduced Inflammation:

Heart disease, diabetes, and some forms of cancer are among the numerous chronic diseases that chronic inflammation is a contributing component to.

The Atkins Diet, which emphasizes whole, nutrient-dense foods and minimizes consumption of processed carbohydrates and inflammatory foods, may help reduce inflammation in the body. By promoting a balanced intake of vitamins, minerals, antioxidants, and phytonutrients, the Atkins Diet supports optimal immune function and cellular repair, potentially reducing the risk of inflammatory-related conditions.

6. Enhanced Physical Performance:
Some proponents of the Atkins Diet claim that it can improve physical performance, particularly in endurance activities, by training the body to rely more efficiently on fat for fuel. In a state of ketosis, which is induced by very low carbohydrate intake, the body produces ketones, which can be used as an alternative fuel source by muscles and the brain. While more research is needed to fully understand the effects of low-carbohydrate diets on athletic performance, some athletes and fitness enthusiasts report benefits such as improved endurance, faster recovery, and reduced muscle fatigue when following a ketogenic or Atkins-style eating plan..

CRITICISM AND CONTROVERSY

Despite its popularity and reported benefits, the Atkins Diet has faced criticism and controversy:

1. Nutritional Imbalance: Critics argue that the Atkins Diet may lack essential nutrients found in whole grains, fruits, and legumes, potentially leading to nutritional deficiencies if not carefully planned.

2. Potential Health Risks: Some experts express concerns about the long-term effects of high-fat diets on heart health, cholesterol levels, and overall mortality, although recent research has challenged these assumptions.

3. Sustainability: Critics question the sustainability and practicality of long-term adherence to a low-carbohydrate eating pattern, especially in the context of social situations and cultural norms.

4. Individual Variation: The effectiveness of the Atkins Diet, like any dietary approach, varies among individuals based on factors such as metabolic health, activity level, genetics, and personal preferences.

HOW TO USE THIS COOKBOOK

Welcome to the Atkins Diet Cookbook 2024! Whether you're new to the Atkins Diet or a seasoned follower looking for fresh recipe ideas, this cookbook is designed to support your journey toward better health, weight loss, and culinary enjoyment. How to maximize this resource is as follows:

1. Understand the Atkins Diet Principles:

Before diving into the recipes, it's essential to familiarize yourself with the principles of the Atkins Diet. As outlined in the introduction, the Atkins Diet is a low-carbohydrate eating plan that emphasizes protein and healthy fats while minimizing intake of carbohydrates, particularly refined sugars and grains. Understanding the four phases of the Atkins Diet—Induction, Balancing, Pre-Maintenance, and Maintenance—will help you navigate the recipes and tailor them to your individual goals and preferences.

2. Choose Recipes That Suit Your Dietary Preferences and Needs:

With a diverse range of recipes spanning breakfast, lunch, dinner, side dishes, snacks, and desserts, this cookbook offers something for everyone. Whether you're a meat lover, a vegetarian, or follow a specific dietary pattern such as keto or paleo, you'll find recipes that align with your preferences and dietary needs. Each recipe is clearly labeled with its nutritional information, including carbohydrate content, making it easy to track your daily intake and stay on target with your goals.

3. Plan Your Meals and Grocery List:

To make meal preparation a breeze, take some time to plan your meals for the week ahead. Browse through the cookbook and select recipes that appeal to you, considering factors such as ingredients on hand, cooking time, and nutritional balance. Once you've chosen your recipes, create a grocery list to ensure you have all the necessary ingredients on hand. Stock up on pantry staples such as oils, spices, and low-carb substitutes like almond flour and coconut oil, so you're always ready to whip up a delicious Atkins-friendly meal.

4. Experiment with Substitutions and Modifications:

Feel free to get creative and experiment with substitutions and modifications to suit your taste preferences and dietary restrictions. Many of the recipes in this cookbook can be customized to accommodate different dietary needs, such as dairy-free, gluten-free, or vegetarian variations. For example, you can swap out dairy ingredients for non-dairy alternatives, use gluten-free flours in place of wheat flour, or incorporate additional vegetables to boost fiber and nutrient content. Don't be afraid to make the recipes your own and tailor them to fit your unique lifestyle and dietary goals.

5. Cook with Confidence and Enjoy the Process:

Cooking should be a fun and rewarding experience, so don't be intimidated by trying new recipes or techniques. Take your time to read through each recipe carefully, gather your ingredients and equipment, and follow the instructions step by step. Cooking can be a creative outlet and an opportunity to nourish your body and soul with delicious, wholesome food. Whether you're cooking for yourself, your family, or friends, savor the experience and take pride in preparing meals that support your health and well-being.

6. Share Your Successes and Discoveries:

As you explore the recipes in this cookbook and embark on your Atkins Diet journey, don't hesitate to share your successes, challenges, and discoveries with others. Join online communities, forums, or social media groups dedicated to the Atkins Diet, where you can connect with like-minded individuals, exchange tips and advice, and celebrate your progress together. Sharing your experiences can be motivating and inspiring, and you may even discover new recipe ideas or cooking techniques along the way.

ESSENTIAL INGREDIENTS FOR ATKINS COOKING

Whether you're just starting your Atkins Diet journey or looking to expand your culinary repertoire, having a well-stocked pantry and fridge is essential for creating delicious, satisfying meals that align with the principles of the Atkins Diet. Here's a comprehensive list of essential ingredients to keep on hand for Atkins cooking:

1. Protein Sources:

Protein is a cornerstone of the Atkins Diet, as it helps promote satiety, preserve lean muscle mass, and support metabolic health. Stock up on a variety of protein-rich foods, including:

- Lean meats such as chicken breast, turkey, pork loin, and lean cuts of beef.
- Fatty fish such as salmon, trout, mackerel, and sardines, which are rich in omega-3 fatty acids.
- Shellfish such as shrimp, crab, and scallops.
- Eggs, which are versatile and can be used in numerous recipes.
- Tofu, tempeh, and other plant-based protein sources for vegetarian options.

2. Healthy Fats:

Contrary to popular belief, fats are not the enemy on the Atkins Diet; they're an essential component of a balanced eating plan. Choose healthy fats that provide essential fatty acids and support overall health, including:

- Avocados, which are rich in monounsaturated fats and fiber.
- For cooking and dressing, use avocado, coconut, and olive oils.
- Nuts and seeds such as almonds, walnuts, chia seeds, and flaxseeds, which are excellent sources of healthy fats and protein.
- Nut butters such as almond butter and peanut butter (choose varieties without added sugars).
- Dairy goods with high fat content, like cream, Greek yogurt, and cheese.

3. Low-Carb Vegetables:

Non-starchy vegetables are an essential component of the Atkins Diet, providing essential vitamins, minerals, fiber, and antioxidants without contributing excessive carbohydrates. Fill your fridge with a colorful array of low-carb vegetables, including:

- Leafy greens such as spinach, kale, Swiss chard, and arugula.
- Cruciferous vegetables such as broccoli, cauliflower, Brussels sprouts, and cabbage.
- Bell peppers, zucchini, eggplant, cucumber, and tomatoes.
- Mushrooms, asparagus, green beans, and snow peas.
- Avocado, which is technically a fruit but is low in carbs and high in healthy fats.

4. Low-Carb Substitutes:

While traditional grains and flours are limited on the Atkins Diet, there are plenty of low-carb substitutes that allow you to enjoy your favorite dishes without sacrificing flavor or texture. Stock up on the following:

- Almond flour, coconut flour, and flaxseed meal for baking and breading.
- Coconut milk, almond milk, or other unsweetened non-dairy milks.
- Low-carb pasta substitutes, like shirataki noodles, spaghetti squash, or zucchini noodles (zoodles).

- Cauliflower rice or broccoli rice as a low-carb alternative to traditional rice.
- Lettuce leaves or collard greens for wrapping sandwiches or making lettuce wraps.

5. Herbs, Spices, and Condiments:

Herbs, spices, and condiments are essential for adding flavor and depth to your Atkins-friendly meals without adding extra carbs or calories. Keep a well-stocked spice rack and fridge with the following:

- Garlic, ginger, onions, and shallots for adding aromatic flavor to dishes.
- Herbs such as basil, parsley, cilantro, thyme, rosemary, and oregano.
- Spices such as cumin, paprika, chili powder, turmeric, cinnamon, and nutmeg.
- Vinegars such as balsamic vinegar, red wine vinegar, apple cider vinegar, and rice vinegar.
- Mustard, hot sauce, sugar-free ketchup, soy sauce (or tamari for gluten-free), and Worcestershire sauce for adding tangy and savory notes.

6. Sugar-Free Sweeteners:

While sugar is off-limits on the Atkins Diet, you can still enjoy sweet treats and desserts by using sugar-free sweeteners that won't spike your blood sugar levels. Opt for natural or artificial sweeteners that are low in carbs and calories, such as:

- Stevia, erythritol, monk fruit extract, or blends of these sweeteners.
- Sugar-free syrups and sauces for adding sweetness to beverages, desserts, and baked goods.
- Unsweetened cocoa powder or sugar-free chocolate chips for satisfying chocolate cravings.

7. Canned and Packaged Goods:

For convenience and versatility, keep a selection of canned and packaged goods on hand for quick and easy meal preparation. Look for options that are low in carbs and free from added sugars, preservatives, and artificial ingredients, including:

- Canned fish such as tuna, salmon, and sardines packed in water or olive oil.
- Canned tomatoes, tomato paste, and tomato sauce (check labels for added sugars).
- Olives, pickles, and marinated artichoke hearts for adding flavor to salads and appetizers.

- Broths and stocks for making soups, stews, and sauces (choose varieties without added sugars or high-carb thickeners).

8. Beverages:

Stay hydrated and satisfied with a selection of low-carb beverages that complement your Atkins Diet lifestyle. Opt for water, herbal tea, and unsweetened coffee as your main hydrating options, and consider adding the following to your drink rotation:

- Sparkling water or club soda for a refreshing, bubbly beverage without added sugars.
- Unsweetened almond milk, coconut milk, or cashew milk for creamy, dairy-free options.
- Sugar-free flavored water enhancers or powdered drink mixes for adding variety to plain water.
- Herbal infusions such as mint, ginger, or chamomile for a calming and flavorful beverage option.

1

BREAKFAST RECIPES

DR. LESLIE J. STEEN

CLASSIC BACON AND EGGS RECIPE

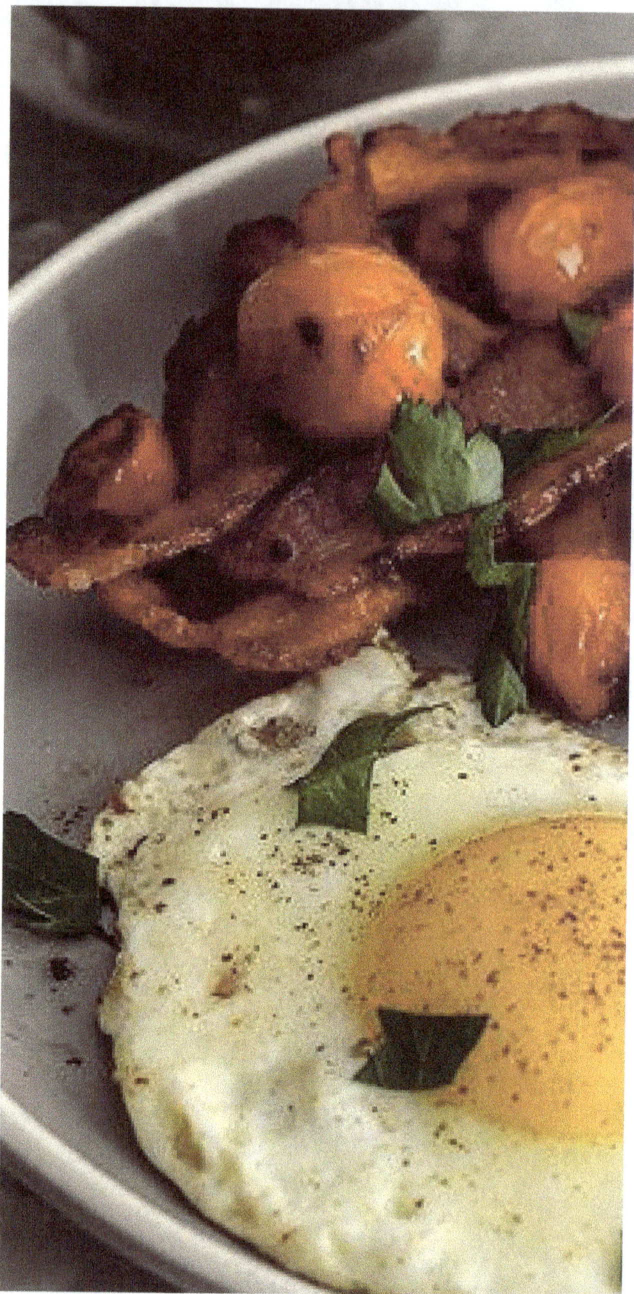

- **Preparation Time** 5 minutes
- **Cooking Time**: 10 minutes
- **Servings**: 2

INGREDIENTS:

- 4 slices of bacon
- 4 large eggs
- Salt and pepper to taste
- Fresh herbs for garnish (optional)

PROCEDURES:

1. Heat a skillet over medium heat and add the bacon slices. Cook the bacon until crisp and golden brown, flipping occasionally to ensure even cooking. This typically takes about 5-7 minutes. After cooking, move the bacon to a dish covered with paper towels so that any leftover fat can be drained.

2. While the bacon is cooking, crack the eggs into a bowl and beat them lightly with a fork or whisk. To taste, add salt and pepper for seasoning.

3. In the same skillet used for cooking the bacon, carefully pour the beaten eggs into the pan. Cook the eggs undisturbed for a minute or two, allowing the edges to set.

4. .Using a spatula, gently push the edges of the eggs towards the center of the pan, allowing the uncooked eggs to flow to the edges. Continue cooking until the eggs are set to your desired consistency, whether you prefer them runny or fully cooked.

5. Once the eggs are cooked to your liking, remove them from the heat and divide them between two plates. Serve the eggs alongside the crispy bacon slices, garnished with fresh herbs if desired.

COOKING TIPS:

- For extra flavor, consider adding a sprinkle of grated cheese or chopped herbs to the beaten eggs before cooking.
- To save time, you can cook the bacon in advance and reheat it briefly in the skillet while cooking the eggs.
- If you prefer your bacon extra crispy, you can bake it in the oven on a foil-lined baking sheet at 400°F (200°C) for about 15-20 minutes, flipping halfway through.

HEALTH BENEFITS:

- Bacon and eggs are rich sources of protein, which is essential for muscle repair, satiety, and overall health.
- Eggs are also packed with essential vitamins and minerals, including vitamin D, vitamin B12, and selenium.
- While bacon is high in saturated fat, it can be part of a balanced diet when enjoyed in moderation and paired with nutrient-rich foods like eggs and vegetables.
- By opting for pastured or organic eggs and nitrate-free bacon, you can minimize your exposure to antibiotics, hormones, and artificial additives.

NUTRITIONAL VALUES (PER SERVING):

- **Calories**: 250
- **Total Fat**: 18g
- **Saturated Fat**: 6g
- **Cholesterol**: 390mg
- **Sodium**: 600mg
- **Total Carbohydrates**: 1g
- **Dietary Fiber**: 0g
- **Sugars**: 0g
- **Protein**: 20g

Note: Nutritional values are approximate and may vary depending on the specific brands and quantities of ingredients used.

SPINACH AND FETA OMELETTE RECIPE

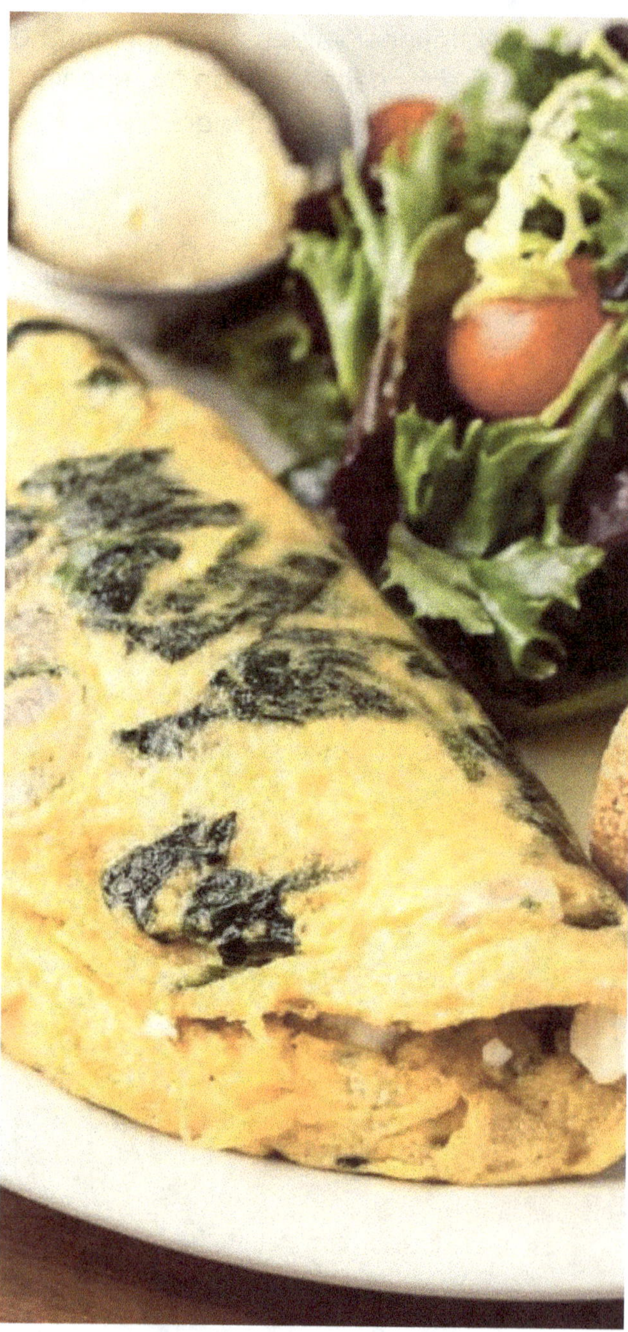

- **Preparation Time**: 5 minutes
- **Cooking Time**: 10 minutes
- **Servings**: 1

INGREDIENTS:

- 2 large eggs
- 1 cup fresh spinach leaves, chopped
- 1/4 cup crumbled feta cheese
- 1 tablespoon olive oil or butter
- Salt and pepper to taste
- Fresh herbs for garnish (optional)

PROCEDURES:

1. In a bowl, crack the eggs and whisk them together until well beaten. To taste, add salt and pepper for seasoning.
2. Heat the olive oil or butter in a non-stick skillet over medium heat. Add the chopped spinach to the skillet and cook for 1-2 minutes, stirring occasionally, until wilted.
3. Pour the beaten eggs over the cooked spinach in the skillet. Let the eggs simmer for a minute or two, or until the edges begin to firm, without moving.
4. Sprinkle the crumbled feta cheese evenly over one half of the omelette.
5. Using a spatula, carefully fold the other half of the omelette over the side with the feta cheese, creating a half-moon shape. Cook for another minute or two, until the eggs are fully cooked and the cheese is melted.
6. Slide the omelette onto a plate and garnish with fresh herbs, if desired. Serve hot and enjoy!

COOKING TIPS:

- Be sure to use a non-stick skillet to prevent the omelette from sticking and facilitate easy flipping.

- Feel free to customize the filling with additional ingredients such as diced tomatoes, sliced mushrooms, or cooked bacon or ham.
- If you prefer a creamier texture, you can add a splash of milk or cream to the beaten eggs before cooking.

HEALTH BENEFITS:

- Eggs are an excellent source of high-quality protein and essential nutrients such as vitamin B12, vitamin D, and choline.
- Spinach is rich in vitamins A, C, and K, as well as iron, magnesium, and antioxidants.
- Feta cheese adds a creamy texture and tangy flavor to the omelette, while also providing calcium and protein.
- Olive oil or butter used for cooking adds healthy fats that are beneficial for heart health and satiety.

NUTRITIONAL VALUES (PER SERVING):

- **Calories**: 330
- **Total Fat**: 26g
- **Saturated Fat**: 9g
- **Cholesterol**: 390mg
- **Sodium**: 630mg
- **Total Carbohydrates**: 4g
- **Dietary Fiber**: 1g
- **Sugars**: 1g
- **Protein**: 20g

Note: Nutritional values are approximate and may vary depending on the specific brands and quantities of ingredients used.

AVOCADO AND BACON BREAKFAST BOWL RECIPE

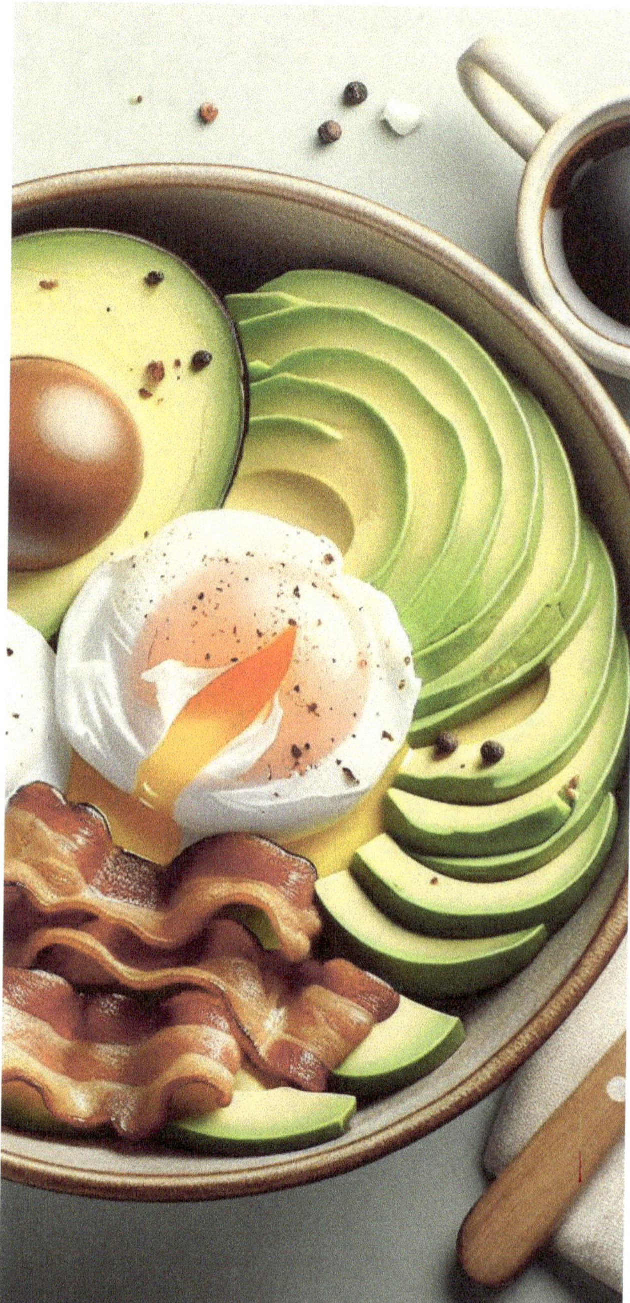

- **Preparation Time:** 10 minutes
- **Cooking Time:** 10 minutes
- **Servings:** 2

INGREDIENTS:

- 2 ripe avocados, halved and pitted
- 4 slices of bacon
- 4 large eggs
- 1 cup cherry tomatoes, halved
- 1/4 cup diced red onion
- 1/4 cup chopped fresh cilantro
- Salt and pepper to taste
- Lime wedges for garnish (optional)

PROCEDURES:

1 Cook the bacon in a skillet over medium heat until crisp and golden brown, about 5-7 minutes. After cooking, move the bacon to a dish covered with paper towels so that any leftover fat can be drained.. Allow to cool slightly, then crumble or chop into bite-sized pieces.

2 While the bacon is cooking, halve and pit the avocados. Use a spoon to scoop out some of the flesh from each avocado half, creating a larger cavity to hold the other ingredients. Keep the avocado flesh that you scooped out for another time.

3 In the same skillet used for cooking the bacon, crack the eggs and cook to your desired level of doneness (e.g., scrambled, fried, or poached). Season with salt and pepper to taste.

4 To assemble the breakfast bowls, place one avocado half in each

serving bowl or plate. Fill the hollowed-out portion of each avocado half with some of the reserved avocado flesh.

5 Divide the cooked bacon, eggs, cherry tomatoes, diced red onion, and chopped cilantro evenly between the avocado halves, arranging them on top of the avocado flesh.

6 Garnish the breakfast bowls with lime wedges, if desired, and serve immediately.

COOKING TIPS:

- For added flavor and texture, consider sprinkling the assembled breakfast bowls with crumbled feta cheese or grated Parmesan cheese.
- To save time, you can cook the bacon and eggs simultaneously in separate skillets, or prepare them in advance and reheat briefly before assembling the breakfast bowls.
- Feel free to customize the ingredients based on your preferences; for example, you can add sliced jalapeños for a spicy kick or diced bell peppers for added color and crunch.

HEALTH BENEFITS:

- Avocados are a nutrient-dense fruit rich in heart-healthy monounsaturated fats, fiber, potassium, and vitamins C, E, and K.
- Bacon and eggs provide high-quality protein and essential nutrients such as vitamin B12, selenium, and choline.
- Cherry tomatoes are packed with antioxidants such as lycopene, as well as vitamins A and C.
- Red onion adds flavor and a dose of antioxidants, including quercetin and sulfur compounds.

NUTRITIONAL VALUES (PER SERVING):

- **Calories**: 400
- **Total Fat**: 30g
- **Saturated** Fat: 6g
- **Cholesterol**: 350mg
- **Sodium**: 420mg
- **Total Carbohydrates**: 15g
- **Dietary Fiber**: 10g
- **Sugars**: 3g
- **Protein**: 20g

Note: Nutritional values are approximate and may vary depending on the specific brands and quantities of ingredients used.

COCONUT FLOUR PANCAKES WITH SUGAR-FREE SYRUP RECIPE

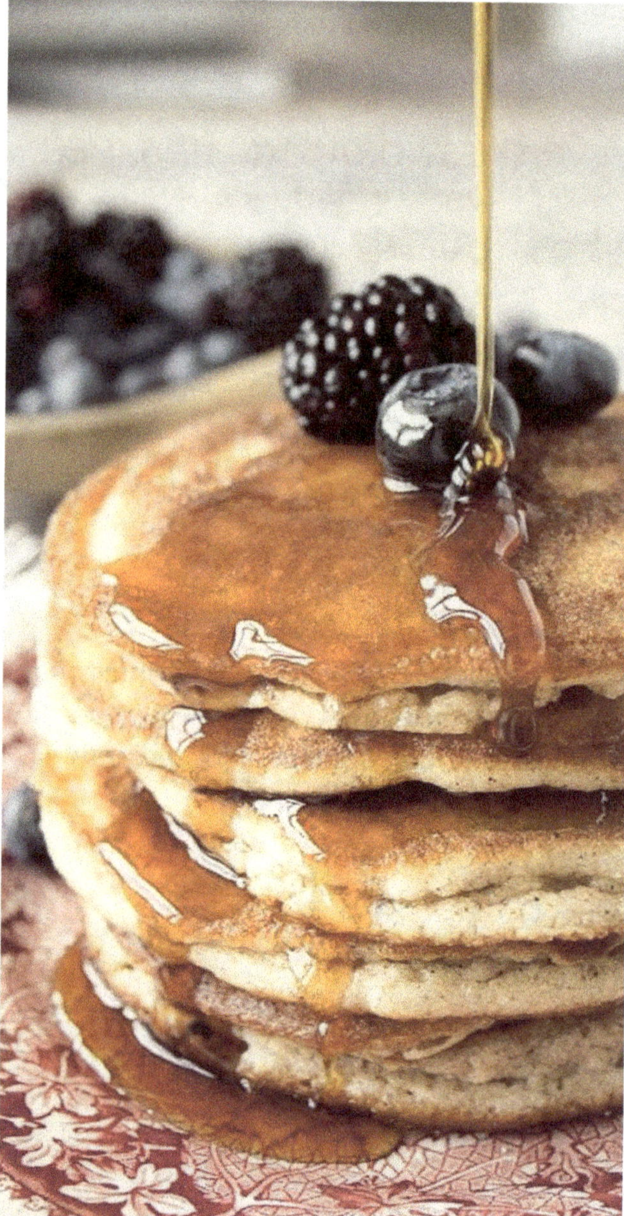

Preparation Time: 10 minutes
Cooking Time: 10 minutes
Servings: 4 (approximately 8 pancakes)

INGREDIENTS

For the pancakes:

- 4 large eggs
- ♣ Half a cup of unsweetened almond milk, or any other type of milk you prefer
- 1/4 cup coconut flour
- 2 tablespoons granulated sweetener of your choice (such as erythritol or stevia)
- 1 teaspoon baking powder
- 1/2 teaspoon vanilla extract
- Pinch of salt
- Coconut oil or butter for cooking

For the sugar-free syrup:

- 1/2 cup water
- 1/4 cup granulated sweetener of your choice
- 1 teaspoon vanilla extract
- Pinch of salt

PROCEDURES:

1. In a large mixing bowl, whisk together the eggs, almond milk, vanilla extract, and sweetener until well combined.
2. In a separate bowl, sift together the coconut flour, baking powder, and salt.
3. Gradually add the dry ingredients to the wet ingredients, stirring until smooth and well incorporated. To let the coconut flour to absorb the liquid, let the batter sit for a few minutes.
4. Heat a non-stick skillet or griddle over medium heat and lightly grease with coconut oil or butter.
5. Spoon about 1/4 cup of batter onto the skillet for each pancake, spreading it out slightly with the back

of the spoon to form a round shape. Cook the pancakes for two to three minutes on each side, or until they are cooked through and golden brown.

6 . While the pancakes are cooking, prepare the sugar-free syrup. In a small saucepan, combine the water, sweetener, vanilla extract, and salt. Bring to a simmer over medium heat, stirring until the sweetener is dissolved. Remove from heat and set aside.

7 Once the pancakes are cooked, stack them on a plate and serve warm with the sugar-free syrup drizzled on top.

COOKING TIPS

- Coconut flour tends to absorb a lot of liquid, so if the batter becomes too thick, you can thin it out with a little extra almond milk.
- Be patient when cooking the pancakes; they may take slightly longer to cook compared to traditional pancakes due to the denser texture of coconut flour.
- To ensure evenly cooked pancakes, make sure the skillet or griddle is preheated properly before adding the batter, and flip the pancakes gently using a spatula.

HEALTH BENEFITS

- Coconut flour is a gluten-free and grain-free alternative to traditional wheat flour, making it suitable for those with gluten sensitivities or following a low-carb diet.
- Coconut flour is rich in fiber, which can help support digestive health, regulate blood sugar levels, and promote satiety.
- Eggs are a nutrient-dense source of high-quality protein, vitamins, and minerals, including vitamin D, vitamin B12, and selenium.
- Unsweetened almond milk is low in calories and carbohydrates, making it a suitable option for those watching their sugar intake.

NUTRITIONAL VALUES (PER SERVING, INCLUDING SYRUP):

- **Calories**: 150
- **Total Fat**: 10g
- **Saturated Fat**: 5g
- **Cholesterol**: 180mg
- **Sodium**: 220mg
- **Total Carbohydrates**: 10g
- **Dietary Fiber**: 4g
- **Sugars**: 1g
- **Protein**: 7g

Note: Nutritional values may vary depending on the specific brands and quantities of ingredients used. Adjustments can be made to the sugar-free syrup recipe to suit individual taste preferences.

SMOKED SALMON AND CREAM CHEESE STUFFED MUSHROOMS RECIPE

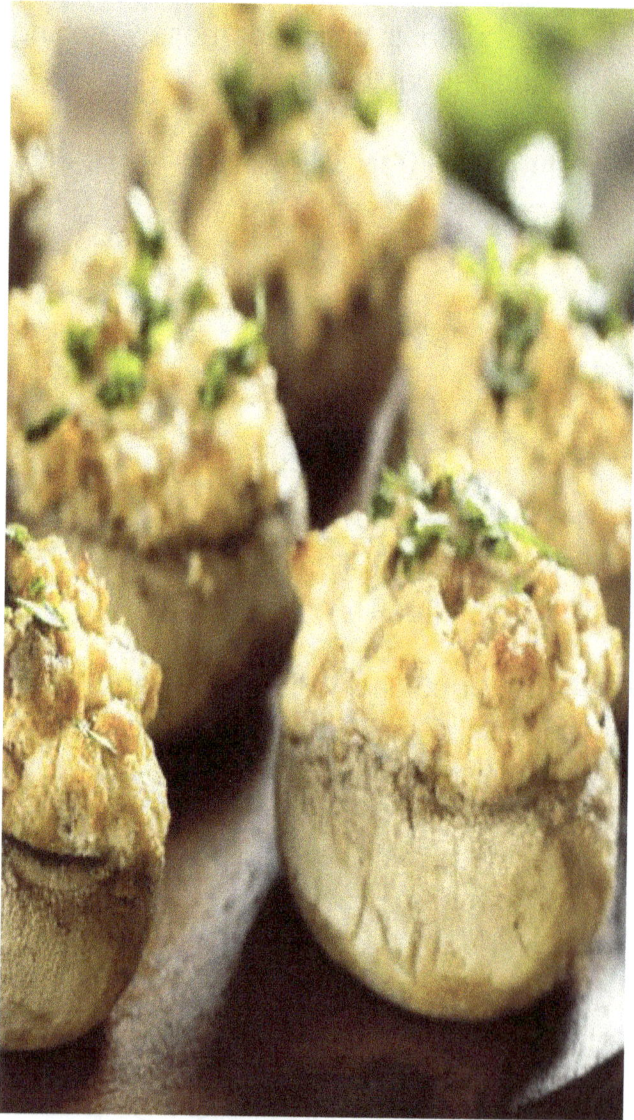

- **Preparation Time**: 15 minutes
- **Cooking Time:** 15 minutes
- **Servings**: 4 (approximately 8 stuffed mushrooms)

INGREDIENTS:

- 16 large mushrooms, stems removed
- 4 ounces smoked salmon, chopped
- 4 ounces cream cheese, softened
- 2 tablespoons finely chopped red onion
- 2 tablespoons chopped fresh dill
- 1 tablespoon lemon juice
- Salt and pepper to taste
- Olive oil for drizzling
- Lemon wedges for serving (optional)

PROCEDURES:

1 Preheat the oven to 375°F (190°C A baking sheet can be lightly oiled with olive oil or lined with parchment paper.
2 To get rid of any dirt, wipe the mushrooms down with a moist towel. Carefully remove the stems from the mushrooms and discard them or reserve for another use.
3 In a mixing bowl, Add salt and pepper to taste, then stir until thoroughly mixed cream cheese, finely chopped red onion, chopped fresh dill, and lemon juice. Season with salt and pepper to taste, and mix until well combined.
4 Spoon the salmon and cream cheese mixture into the cavity of each mushroom, filling them generously.
5 Put the filled mushrooms onto the baking sheet that has been ready. Drizzle with olive oil and sprinkle with additional chopped dill, if desired.

6 Bake in the preheated oven for 12-15 minutes, or until the mushrooms are tender and the filling is heated through and slightly golden on top.

7 7. Take out of the oven and allow it to cool down a little before serving. Serve the stuffed mushrooms warm, garnished with lemon wedges if desired.

COOKING TIPS:

- Choose large mushrooms with firm caps to hold the filling without collapsing during baking.
- To make the cream cheese easier to work with, let it soften at room temperature for about 30 minutes before mixing with the other ingredients.
- Feel free to customize the filling by adding ingredients such as minced garlic, capers, or chopped fresh parsley for extra flavor.
- If you prefer a crispy topping, you can sprinkle the stuffed mushrooms with breadcrumbs or grated Parmesan cheese before baking.

- Mushrooms are low in calories and carbohydrates, making them a suitable option for those following a low-carb or keto diet.
- Smoked salmon is rich in omega-3 fatty acids, which are beneficial for heart health and brain function.
- Cream cheese provides a creamy texture and adds richness to the filling, while also providing calcium and protein.
- Dill and lemon juice add bright, refreshing flavors to the dish and provide antioxidants and vitamins.

NUTRITIONAL VALUES (PER SERVING):

- **Calories**: 140
- **Total Fat**: 10g
- **Saturated Fat**: 5g
- **Cholesterol**: 30mg
- **Sodium**: 220mg
- **Total Carbohydrates**: 4g
- **Dietary Fiber**: 1g
- **Sugars**: 2g
- **Protein**: 9g

NOTE: Nutritional values are approximate and may vary depending on the specific brands and quantities of ingredients used.

HEALTH BENEFITS:

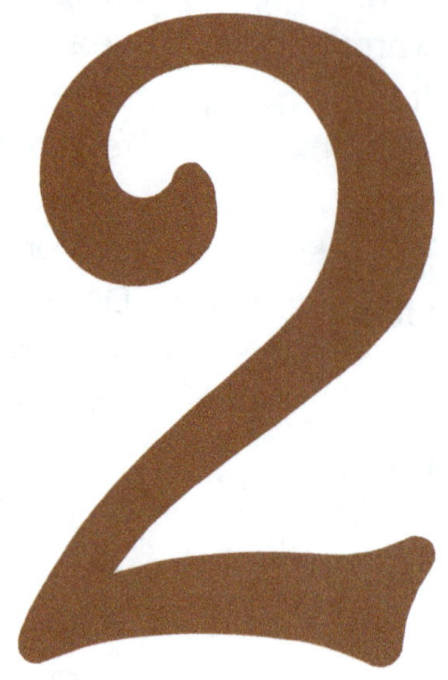

2

LUNCH RECIPES

DR. LESLIE J. STEEN

GRILLED CHICKEN CAESAR SALAD RECIPE

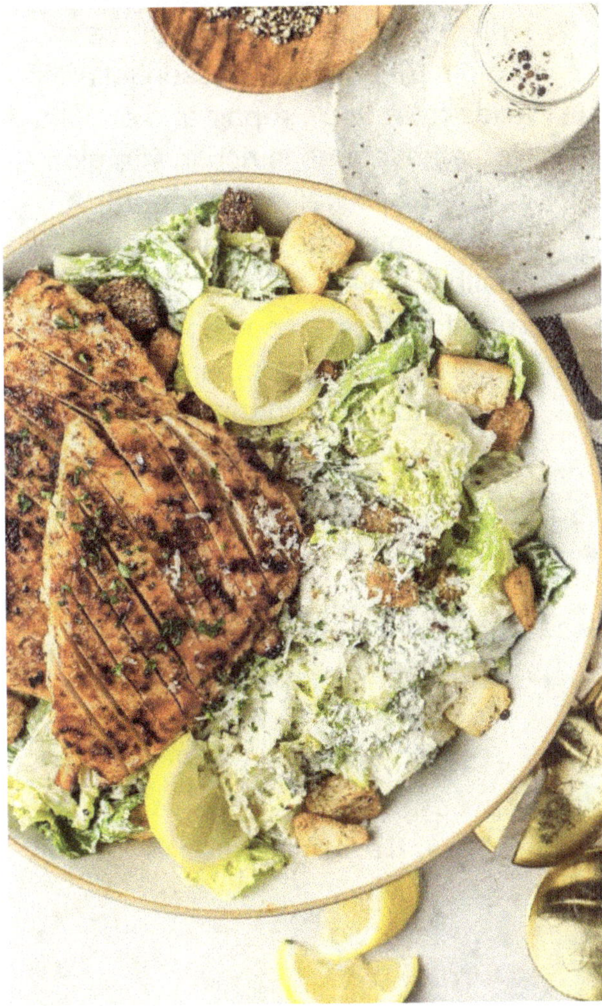

- **Preparation Time**: 15 minutes
- **Cooking Time**: 15 minutes
- **Servings**: 4

INGREDIENTS:

For the grilled chicken:
- 4 boneless, skinless chicken breasts
- 2 tablespoons olive oil
- 2 cloves garlic, minced
- 1 teaspoon dried oregano
- 1 teaspoon dried thyme
- Salt and pepper to taste

For the Caesar dressing:
- 1/2 cup mayonnaise
- 2 tablespoons grated Parmesan cheese
- 1 tablespoon lemon juice
- 1 teaspoon Dijon mustard
- 1 clove garlic, minced
- Salt and pepper to taste

For the salad:
- 1 large head of romaine lettuce, chopped
- 1 cup cherry tomatoes, halved
- 1/2 cup croutons (optional)
- Additional grated Parmesan cheese for garnish

PROCEDURES:

1 Preheat the grill to medium-high heat.

2 In a small bowl, whisk together the olive oil, minced garlic, dried oregano, dried thyme, salt, and pepper to make the marinade for the chicken.

3 Place the chicken breasts in a shallow dish or resealable plastic bag. Pour the marinade over the chicken, making sure to coat each breast evenly. Allow the chicken to marinate for at least 15 minutes, or up to 1 hour in the refrigerator.

4 While the chicken is marinating, prepare the Caesar dressing Combine the mayonnaise, lemon juice, Dijon mustard, grated Parmesan cheese, minced garlic, salt, and pepper in a mixing bowl. Whisk until smooth and well combined. Adjust the seasoning to

taste, adding more lemon juice or Parmesan cheese if desired. Set aside.

5   Once the grill is preheated, remove the chicken from the marinade and discard any excess marinade. Place the chicken breasts on the grill and cook for 6-8 minutes per side, or until cooked through and no longer pink in the center. The internal temperature should reach 165°F (75°C Before slicing, take the chicken off the grill and let it a few minutes to rest.

6   6 Make the salad while the chicken is resting. In a large mixing bowl, combine the chopped romaine lettuce, halved cherry tomatoes, and croutons (if using). Toss the salad with the prepared Caesar dressing until evenly coated.

7   To serve, divide the dressed salad among serving plates. Top each salad with slices of grilled chicken and garnish with additional grated Parmesan cheese, if desired. Serve immediately and enjoy!

COOKING TIPS:

- To ensure juicy and flavorful grilled chicken, avoid overcooking. Use a meat thermometer to check for doneness, and remove the chicken from the grill once it reaches an internal temperature of 165°F (75°C).
- If you prefer, you can use store-bought Caesar dressing instead of making it from scratch Choose products that have the fewest artificial additives and added sugars possible.

- For added flavor and texture, consider adding other salad toppings such as sliced cucumbers, avocado, or hard-boiled eggs.

HEALTH BENEFITS:

- Grilled chicken is a lean source of protein that provides essential amino acids for muscle repair and growth.
- Romaine lettuce is rich in vitamins A, C, and K, as well as fiber and antioxidants that support overall health and well-being.
- Tomatoes are a good source of vitamin C, potassium, and lycopene, a powerful antioxidant with potential health benefits.

NUTRITIONAL VALUES (PER SERVING):

- **Calories**: 350
- **Total Fat**: 20g
- **Saturated Fat**: 4g
- **Cholesterol**: 90mg
- **Sodium**: 450mg
- **Total Carbohydrates**: 10g
- **Dietary Fiber**: 3g
- **Sugars**: 3g
- **Protein**: 30g

TURKEY AND AVOCADO LETTUCE WRAPS RECIPE

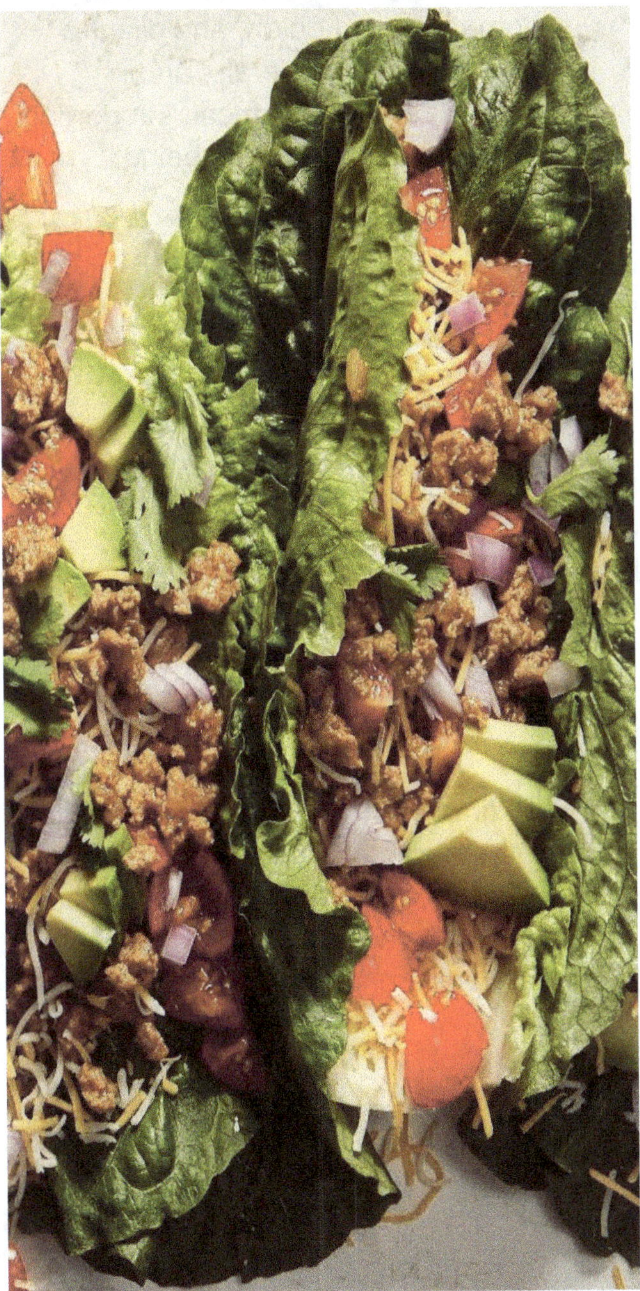

- **Preparation Time**: 15 minutes
- **Cooking Time**: 10 minutes
- **Servings**: 4

INGREDIENTS:

- 1 lb (450g) ground turkey
- 2 tablespoons olive oil
- 2 cloves garlic, minced
- 1 teaspoon ground cumin
- 1 teaspoon chili powder
- 1/2 teaspoon paprika
- Salt and pepper to taste
- 1 large avocado, diced
- 1/2 cup cherry tomatoes, diced
- 1/4 cup red onion, finely chopped
- 1/4 cup fresh cilantro, chopped
- Juice of 1 lime
- Large lettuce leaves, such butter or romaine, are an optional topping. You can also add shredded cheese, sour cream, or salsa.

PROCEDURES:

1. Heat olive oil in a skillet over medium heat. Add minced garlic and sauté until fragrant, about 1 minute.
2. Add ground turkey to the skillet, breaking it up with a spatula. Cook until turkey is browned and cooked through, about 5-7 minutes.
3. Stir in ground cumin, chili powder, paprika, salt, and pepper. Simmer for a further two to three minutes to let the flavors combine.
4. Remove the skillet from heat and transfer the cooked turkey to a large mixing bowl. Let it cool slightly.
5. Add diced avocado, cherry tomatoes, red onion, fresh cilantro, and lime juice to the bowl with the cooked turkey. Gently toss to combine.
6. To assemble the lettuce wraps, place a spoonful of the turkey and

avocado mixture onto each lettuce leaf. Roll up the lettuce leaf around the filling, securing it with a toothpick if necessary.

7 Serve the turkey and avocado lettuce wraps immediately, garnished with additional cilantro and lime wedges if desired. Offer optional toppings such as salsa, sour cream, or shredded cheese for added flavor.

COOKING TIPS:

- Choose lean ground turkey for a healthier option with less saturated fat.
- You are welcome to modify the seasonings according to your personal tastes.
- . Add more chili powder for extra heat or sprinkle with a pinch of cayenne pepper.
- For a time-saving option, you can use leftover cooked turkey or chicken instead of cooking ground turkey from scratch.
- To make the lettuce wraps more filling, you can add additional fillings such as cooked quinoa, black beans, or diced bell peppers.

HEALTH BENEFITS:

- Turkey is a lean source of protein that provides essential amino acids for muscle repair and growth.
- Avocado is rich in heart-healthy monounsaturated fats, fiber, and potassium, which may help lower cholesterol levels and reduce the risk of heart disease.

- Lettuce leaves are low in calories and carbohydrates, making them an excellent alternative to traditional tortillas for those following a low-carb diet.
- Fresh vegetables such as cherry tomatoes, red onion, and cilantro add vitamins, minerals, and antioxidants to the meal, supporting overall health and well-being.

NUTRITIONAL VALUES (PER SERVING, 2 LETTUCE WRAPS):

- Calories: 250
- Total Fat: 15g
- Saturated Fat: 3g
- Cholesterol: 60mg
- Sodium: 250mg
- Total Carbohydrates: 10g
- Dietary Fiber: 5g
- Sugars: 2g
- Protein: 20g

NOTE: Nutritional values are approximate and may vary depending on the specific brands and quantities of ingredients used. Adjustments can be made to the recipe to suit individual dietary preferences and requirements.

TUNA Salad Stuffed Bell Peppers Recipe

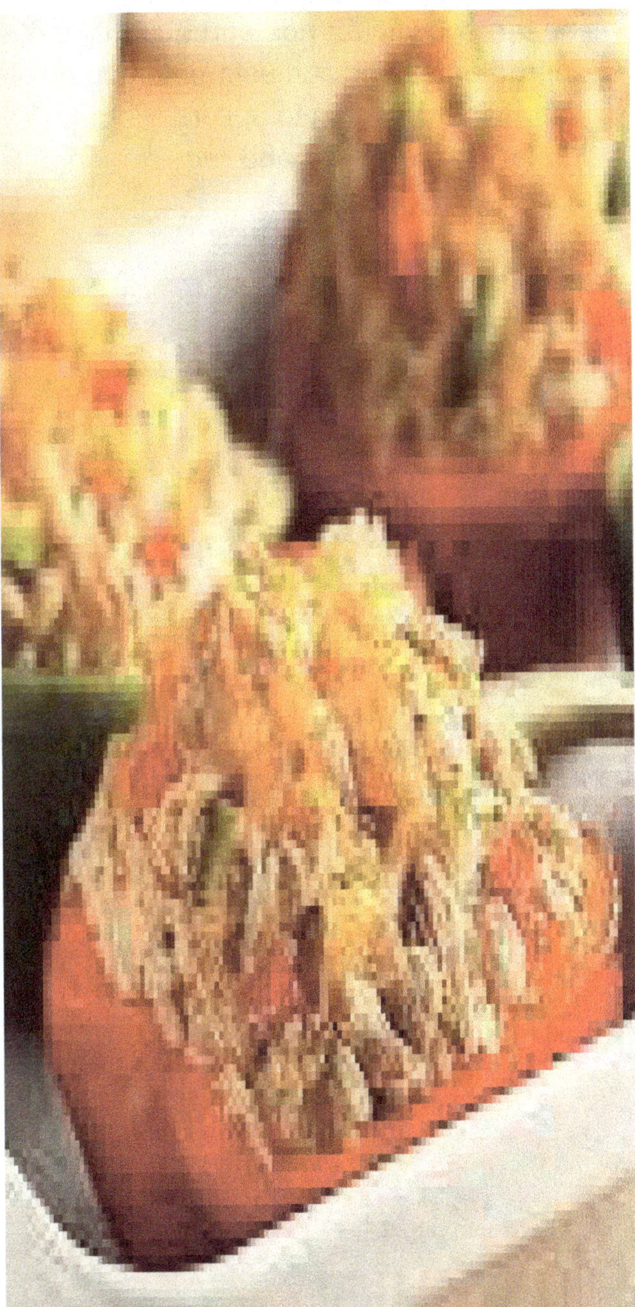

- **Preparation Time**: 15 minutes
- **Cooking Time**: 0 minutes
- **Servings**: 4

INGREDIENTS:

- 4 large bell peppers, any color
- Two drained cans (5 ounces each) of tuna
- 1/2 cup mayonnaise
- 1/4 cup diced red onion
- 1/4 cup diced celery
- 2 tablespoons chopped fresh parsley
- 1 tablespoon lemon juice
- 1 teaspoon Dijon mustard
- Salt and pepper to taste
- Optional toppings: sliced cherry tomatoes, sliced olives, shredded cheese

PROCEDURES:

1. Slice the tops off the bell peppers and remove the seeds and membranes. Cut a small slice from the bottom of each pepper to create a flat surface, allowing them to stand upright.
2. In a large mixing bowl, combine the drained tuna, mayonnaise, diced red onion, diced celery, chopped fresh parsley, lemon juice, Dijon mustard, salt, and pepper. Stir thoroughly to ensure that all ingredients are combined equally.
3. Spoon the tuna salad mixture into each bell pepper, filling them to the top and pressing down gently to pack the filling.
4. If desired, top each stuffed bell pepper with sliced cherry tomatoes, sliced olives, or shredded cheese for extra flavor and presentation.
5. Serve the tuna salad stuffed bell peppers immediately, or refrigerate until ready to serve.

COOKING TIPS:

- Choose firm, evenly-shaped bell peppers with flat bottoms for stability when standing upright.
- For added crunch and flavor, you can mix in additional ingredients such as diced cucumber, grated carrot, or chopped pickles.
- To save time, you can use pre-cooked or canned tuna instead of cooking fresh tuna.

HEALTH BENEFITS:

- Bell peppers are rich in vitamins A and C, antioxidants, and fiber, which support immune function, skin health, and digestion.
- Tuna is a lean source of protein that provides essential amino acids for muscle repair and growth.
- Celery and red onion add crunch and flavor to the tuna salad while also providing vitamins, minerals, and antioxidants.
- Parsley is a nutrient-dense herb that adds freshness and color to the dish, as well as vitamins A, C, and K.

NUTRITIONAL VALUES (PER SERVING, 1 STUFFED BELL PEPPER):

- **Calories**: 250
- **Total Fat**: 15g
- **Saturated Fat**: 2g
- **Cholesterol**: 40mg
- **Sodium**: 500mg
- **Total Carbohydrates**: 10g
- **Dietary Fiber**: 3g
- **Sugars**: 5g
- **Protein**: 20g

NOTE: Nutritional values are approximate and may vary depending on the specific brands and quantities of ingredients used. Adjustments can be made to the recipe to suit individual dietary preferences and requirements.

ZUCCHINI NOODLES WITH PESTO AND CHERRY TOMATOES RECIPE

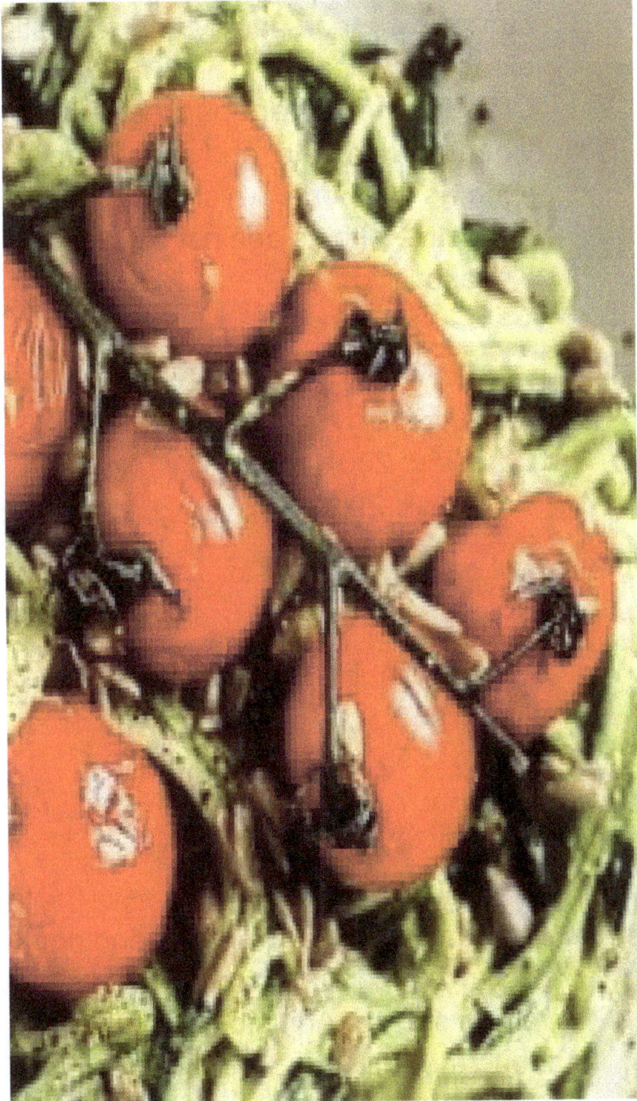

- **Preparation Time:** 15 minutes
- **Cooking Time:** 10 minutes
- **Servings**: 4

INGREDIENTS:

For the zucchini noodles:

- 4 medium zucchini
- 2 tablespoons olive oil
- Salt and pepper to taste

For the pesto:

- 2 cups fresh basil leaves, packed
- 1/4 cup pine nuts or walnuts
- 2 cloves garlic, minced
- 1/2 cup grated Parmesan cheese
- 1/4 cup olive oil
- Salt and pepper to taste

For serving:

- 1 cup cherry tomatoes, halved
- Additional grated Parmesan cheese for garnish
- Fresh basil leaves for garnish

PROCEDURES:

1 Using a spiralizer or vegetable peeler, create zucchini noodles by slicing the zucchini into thin strips resembling spaghetti. Set aside.

2 In a food processor or blender, combine the basil leaves, pine nuts or walnuts, minced garlic, grated Parmesan cheese, olive oil, salt, and pepper. Pulse until the ingredients are finely chopped and well combined, forming a smooth pesto sauce.

3 In a big skillet over medium heat, warm up the olive oil. When the zucchini noodles are just soft, add them to the skillet and cook, stirring periodically, for two to three minutes. They can get mushy if you overcook them, so take caution.

4 Once the zucchini noodles are cooked, add the cherry tomatoes to the skillet and toss to combine. Cook for an additional 1-2 minutes, just

until the tomatoes are heated through but still firm.

5   Remove the skillet from heat and stir in the prepared pesto sauce, tossing gently to coat the zucchini noodles and cherry tomatoes evenly.

6   To serve, divide the zucchini noodles and cherry tomatoes among serving plates. If preferred, garnish with more grated Parmesan cheese and fresh basil leaves.

COOKING TIPS:

- If you don't have a spiralizer, you can use a julienne peeler or mandoline slicer to create zucchini noodles, or even purchase pre-packaged zucchini noodles from the store for convenience.
- Toasting the pine nuts or walnuts before adding them to the pesto can enhance their flavor. Simply heat them in a dry skillet over medium heat for a few minutes, stirring occasionally, until golden brown and fragrant.
- For a creamier pesto sauce, you can add a splash of heavy cream or Greek yogurt to the blender when combining the other ingredients.

HEALTH BENEFITS:

- Zucchini is low in calories and carbohydrates, making it an excellent alternative to traditional pasta for those following a low-carb or keto diet. In addition, it contains plenty of fiber, vitamins, and minerals.
- Basil is rich in antioxidants and essential oils that may help reduce inflammation and promote heart health.
- Pine nuts and walnuts provide healthy fats, protein, and fiber, which can help support satiety and regulate blood sugar levels.
- Cherry tomatoes are packed with vitamins, minerals, and antioxidants such as lycopene, which may have protective effects against certain diseases.

NUTRITIONAL VALUES (PER SERVING):

- **Calories**: 250
- **Total Fat**: 20g
- **Saturated Fat**: 4g
- **Cholesterol**: 5mg
- **Sodium**: 200mg
- **Total Carbohydrates**: 10g
- **Dietary Fiber**: 4g
- **Sugars**: 5g
- **Protein**: 7g

NOTE: Nutritional values are approximate and may vary depending on the specific brands and quantities of ingredients used. Adjustments can be made to the recipe to suit individual dietary preferences and requirements.

KETO-FRIENDLY BROCCOLI CHEDDAR SOUP RECIPE

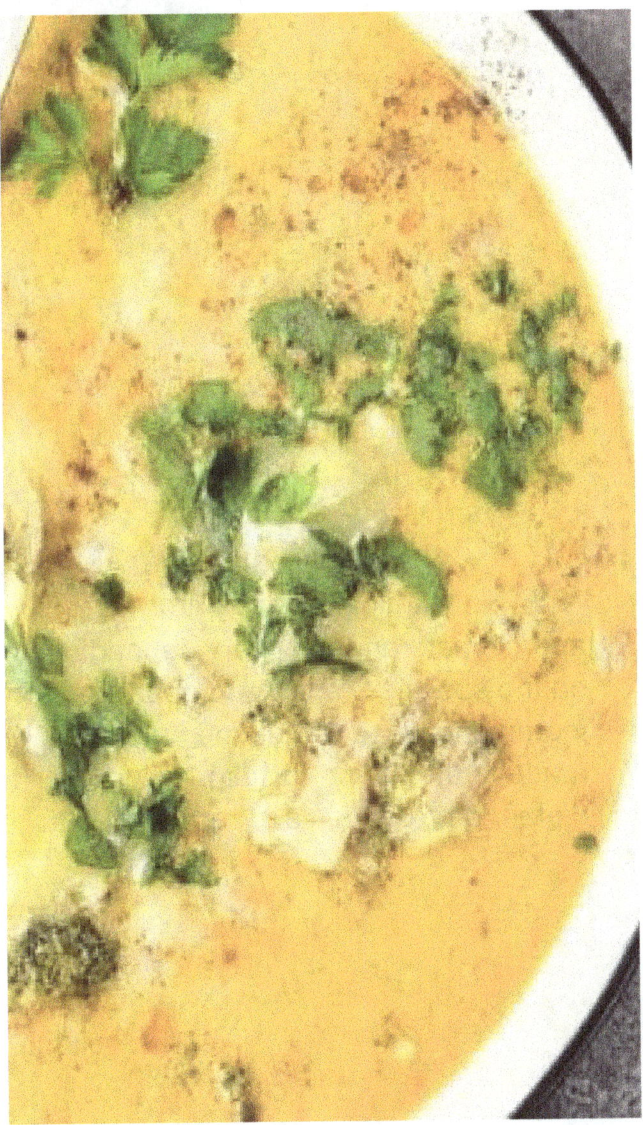

- **Preparation Time**: 10 minutes
- **Cooking Time**: 25 minutes
- **Servings**: 4

INGREDIENTS:

- 4 cups fresh broccoli florets
- 2 tablespoons butter or olive oil
- 1/2 cup diced onion
- 2 cloves garlic, minced
- 4 cups chicken or vegetable broth
- 1 cup heavy cream
- 2 cups shredded cheddar cheese
- Salt and pepper to taste
- Optional toppings: additional shredded cheddar cheese, cooked bacon bits, chopped green onions

PROCEDURES:

1. In a large pot or Dutch oven, melt the butter or heat the olive oil over medium heat. Add the minced garlic and chopped onion, and sauté for two to three minutes, or until aromatic and softened.
2. Add the broccoli florets to the pot and cook for another 3-4 minutes, stirring occasionally, until the broccoli is bright green and slightly tender.
3. Pour the chicken or vegetable broth into the pot and bring to a simmer. Cover and cook for 10-12 minutes, or until the broccoli is tender.
4. Use an immersion blender or transfer the soup to a blender in batches to puree until smooth. Be cautious when blending hot liquids.
5. Return the pureed soup to the pot over low heat. Stir in the heavy cream and shredded cheddar cheese until the cheese is melted and the soup is creamy and smooth.

6 6 Add salt and pepper to taste and season the soup. Adjust the seasoning as needed.

7 Serve the keto-friendly broccoli cheddar soup hot, garnished with additional shredded cheddar cheese, cooked bacon bits, and chopped green onions if desired.

COOKING TIPS:

- For added texture and flavor, reserve a handful of broccoli florets before pureeing the soup and stir them back into the pot before serving.
- To make the soup thicker, you can simmer it uncovered over low heat for a few additional minutes to allow some of the liquid to evaporate.
- If you prefer a smoother soup, you can strain it through a fine mesh sieve after pureeing to remove any remaining solids.

HEALTH BENEFITS:

- Broccoli is a nutrient-dense vegetable rich in vitamins C, K, and folate, as well as fiber and antioxidants that support immune function and overall health.
- Cheddar cheese provides calcium, protein, and healthy fats, which can help promote satiety and support bone health.
- Olive oil and heavy cream add richness and flavor to the soup while providing essential fatty acids and energy.

NUTRITIONAL VALUES (PER SERVING):

- **Calories**: 400
- **Total Fat**: 30g
- **Saturated Fat**: 18g
- **Cholesterol**: 90mg
- **Sodium**: 800mg
- **Total Carbohydrates**: 10g
- **Dietary Fiber**: 2g
- **Sugars**: 4g
- **Protein**: 15g

NOTE: Nutritional values are approximate and may vary depending on the specific brands and quantities of ingredients used. Adjustments can be made to the recipe to suit individual dietary preferences and requirements.

3

DINNER RECIPES

DR. LESLIE J. STEEN

GARLIC BUTTER STEAK BITES RECIPE

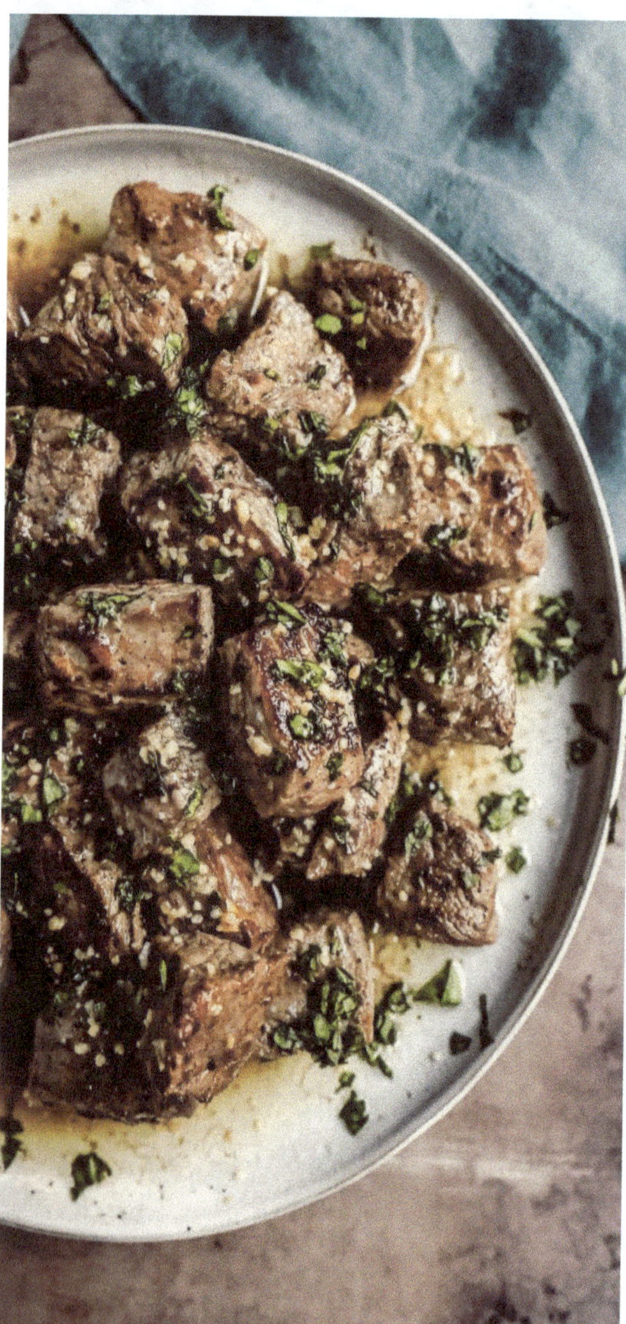

- **Preparation Time**: 10 minutes
- **Cooking Time**: 10 minutes
- **Servings**: 4

INGREDIENTS

- 1 lb (450g) beef sirloin steak, cut into bite-sized pieces
- 2 tablespoons butter
- 4 cloves garlic, minced
- 1 tablespoon soy sauce or Worcestershire sauce
- Salt and pepper to taste
- Chopped fresh parsley for garnish (optional)

PROCEDURES

1. Season the bite-sized steak pieces with salt and pepper on all sides.
2. Heat a large skillet over medium-high heat to melt the butter. When the garlic is fragrant, add it to the skillet and sauté it for one to two minutes.
3. Add the seasoned steak pieces to the skillet in a single layer, making sure not to overcrowd the pan. Cook the steak for 2-3 minutes per side, or until browned and cooked to your desired level of doneness.
4. Once the steak is cooked, drizzle soy sauce or Worcestershire sauce over the steak in the skillet. Toss the steak bites in the sauce until evenly coated.
5. Remove the skillet from heat and transfer the garlic butter steak bites to a serving platter. If desired, garnish with freshly chopped parsley.
6. Serve the garlic butter steak bites hot as a delicious appetizer, main dish, or topping for salads and pasta dishes.

COOKING TIPS:

- For best results, use a high-quality cut of beef such as sirloin, ribeye, or filet mignon for tender and flavorful steak bites.
- Allow the steak to come to room temperature for about 30 minutes before cooking to ensure even cooking and optimal flavor.
- Be careful not to overcook the steak bites, as they can become tough and chewy. Cook them just until they reach your desired level of doneness.
- For a richer flavor, you can add a splash of red wine or balsamic vinegar to the skillet along with the soy sauce or Worcestershire sauce.

HEALTH BENEFITS

- Beef is a good source of high-quality protein, iron, zinc, and B vitamins, which are essential for muscle repair, energy production, and overall health.
- Garlic contains sulfur compounds and antioxidants that may help boost immune function, reduce inflammation, and support heart health.
- Butter adds richness and flavor to the dish, while also providing essential fatty acids and fat-soluble vitamins such as vitamin A and vitamin E.

NUTRITIONAL VALUES (PER SERVING):

- **Calories**: 250
- **Total Fat**: 15g
- **Saturated Fat**: 7g
- **Cholesterol**: 80mg
- **Sodium**: 300mg
- **Total Carbohydrates**: 1g
- **Dietary Fiber**: 0g
- **Sugars**: 0g
- **Protein**: 25g

NOTE: Nutritional values are approximate and may vary depending on the specific brands and quantities of ingredients used. Adjustments can be made to the recipe to suit individual dietary preferences and requirements.

BAKED LEMON HERB SALMON RECIPE

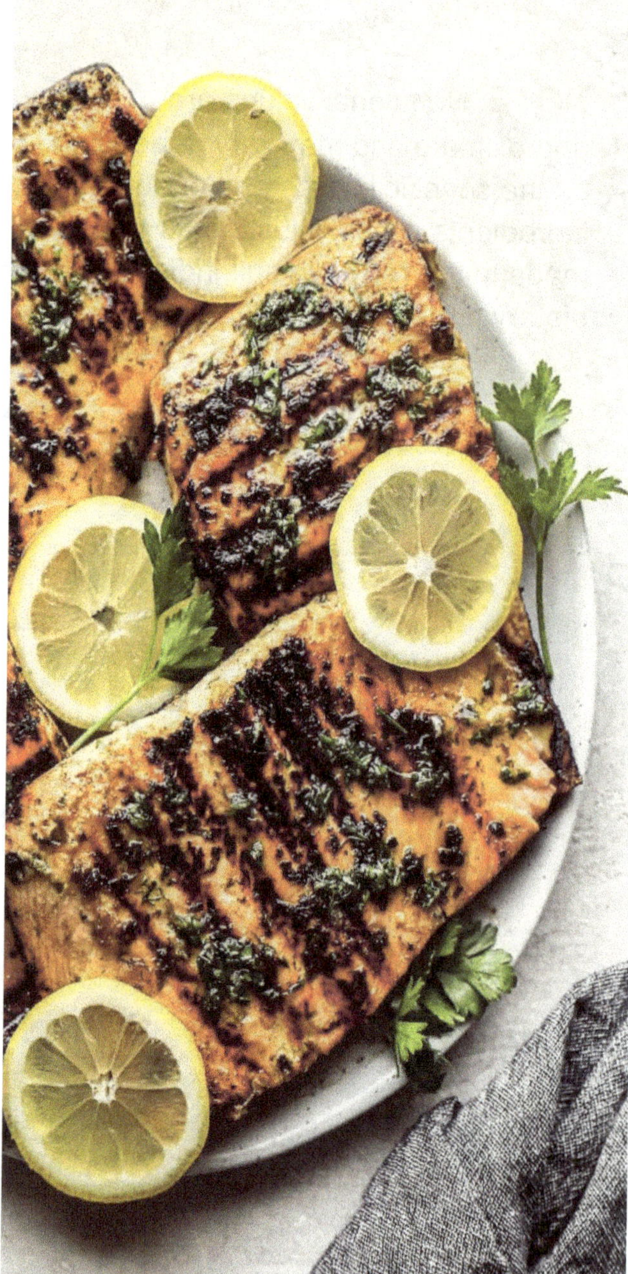

Preparation Time: 10 minutes
Cooking Time: 15 minutes
Servings: 4

INGREDIENTS:

- 4 salmon fillets, about 6 ounces each
- 2 tablespoons olive oil
- 2 cloves garlic, minced
- 1 tablespoon fresh lemon juice
- 1 teaspoon lemon zest
- 1 teaspoon chopped fresh parsley
- 1 teaspoon chopped fresh dill
- Salt and pepper to taste
- Lemon slices for garnish

PROCEDURES:

1. Preheat the oven to 400°F (200°C). A baking sheet can be lightly oiled with olive oil or lined with parchment paper.
2. In a small bowl, whisk together the olive oil, minced garlic, lemon juice, lemon zest, chopped parsley, chopped dill, salt, and pepper to create the herb marinade.
3. Place the salmon fillets on the prepared baking sheet, skin-side down. Brush the herb marinade generously over the top of each salmon fillet, coating them evenly.
4. Arrange lemon slices on top of each salmon fillet for added flavor and presentation.
5. Bake the salmon in the preheated oven for 12-15 minutes, or until the fish is opaque and flakes easily with a fork. The internal temperature of the salmon should reach 145°F (63°C) to ensure it is fully cooked.
6. Once the salmon is cooked, remove it from the oven and let it rest for a few minutes before serving.
7. Serve the baked lemon herb salmon hot, garnished with additional

chopped fresh herbs and lemon wedges if desired.

COOKING TIPS:

- Select premium, fresh salmon fillets for optimal flavor and texture. Look for fillets that are firm and shiny with no strong odor.
- To prevent the salmon from sticking to the baking sheet, you can place the fillets on a bed of lemon slices or parchment paper before baking.
- For added flavor, you can sprinkle the salmon fillets with a pinch of your favorite herbs and spices before baking, such as smoked paprika, thyme, or rosemary.
- Be cautious not to overcook the salmon, as it can become dry and less flavorful. Check for doneness by gently inserting a fork into the thickest part of the fillet; the flesh should flake easily and be opaque throughout.

HEALTH BENEFITS

- Salmon is rich in omega-3 fatty acids, which have been linked to numerous health benefits, including reduced inflammation, improved heart health, and brain function.
- Garlic contains sulfur compounds with potential antimicrobial and immune-boosting properties, as well as antioxidants that may help protect against chronic diseases.
- Fresh herbs like parsley and dill are packed with vitamins, minerals, and antioxidants that support overall health and well-being.

NUTRITIONAL VALUES (PER SERVING):

- **Calories**: 300
- **Total Fat**: 20g
- **Saturated Fat**: 3g
- **Cholesterol**: 80mg
- **Sodium**: 100mg
- **Total Carbohydrates**: 1g
- **Dietary Fiber**: 0g
- **Sugars**: 0g
- **Protein**: 25g

NOTE: Nutritional values are approximate and may vary depending on the specific brands and quantities of ingredients used. Adjustments can be made to the recipe to suit individual dietary preferences and requirements.

CAULIFLOWER CRUST PIZZA WITH PEPPERONI AND MUSHROOMS RECIPE

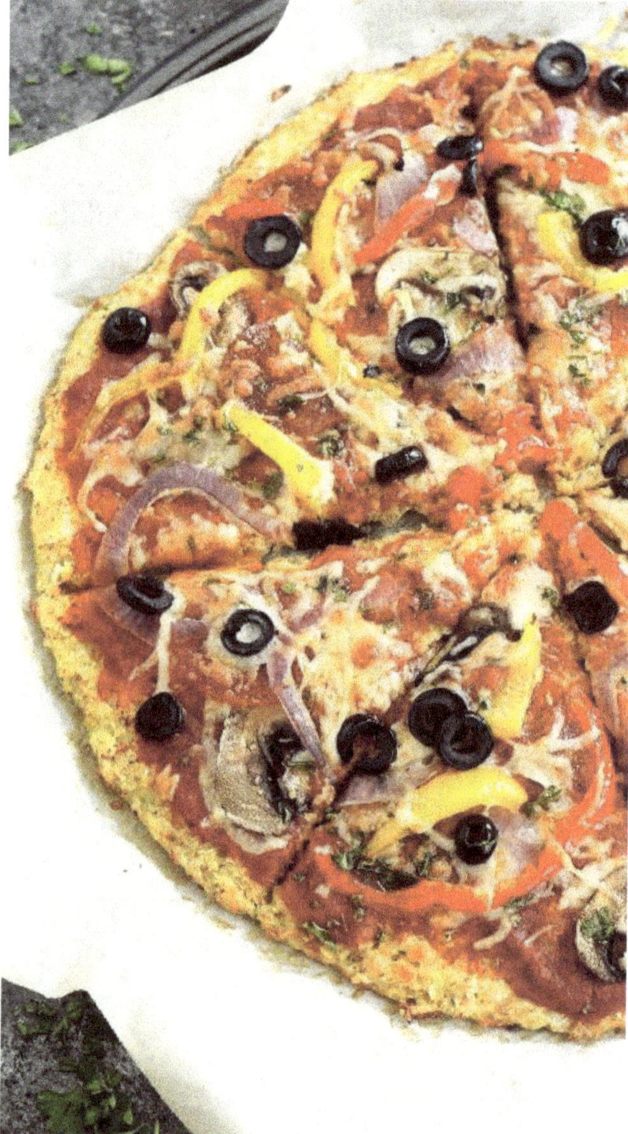

- **Preparation Time:** 20 minutes
- **Cooking Time**: 25 minutes
- **Servings**: 4

INGREDIENTS

For the cauliflower crust:

- 1 medium head cauliflower, cut into florets
- 1/2 cup shredded mozzarella cheese
- 1/4 cup grated Parmesan cheese
- 1 teaspoon dried oregano
- 1/2 teaspoon garlic powder
- 1/4 teaspoon salt
- 1/4 teaspoon black pepper
- 1 large egg, lightly beaten

For the pizza toppings:

- 1/2 cup pizza sauce or marinara sauce
- 1 cup shredded mozzarella cheese
- 1/2 cup sliced pepperoni
- 1/2 cup sliced mushrooms
- Fresh basil leaves for garnish (optional)

PROCEDURES:

1. Preheat the oven to 425°F (220°C). Use parchment paper to line a baking sheet.
2. Place the cauliflower florets in a food processor and pulse until they resemble fine crumbs, resembling rice.
3. Transfer the cauliflower crumbs to a microwave-safe bowl and microwave on high for 4-5 minutes, or until softened. Give it a few minutes to cool.
4. Place the softened cauliflower in a clean kitchen towel or cheesecloth and squeeze out as much moisture as possible. This step is crucial to ensure a crispy cauliflower crust.
5. In a large mixing bowl, combine the squeezed cauliflower, shredded

mozzarella cheese, grated Parmesan cheese, dried oregano, garlic powder, salt, black pepper, and beaten egg. Mix until well combined and a dough-like consistency forms.

6 Transfer the cauliflower dough to the prepared baking sheet and shape it into a round pizza crust, about 1/4 inch thick. Bake in the preheated oven for 15-18 minutes, or until the crust is golden brown and firm to the touch.

7 Take the cauliflower crust out of the oven and evenly coat it with pizza sauce.

8 . Sprinkle shredded mozzarella cheese on top, followed by sliced pepperoni and mushrooms.

9 Return the pizza to the oven and bake for an additional 8-10 minutes, or until the cheese is melted and bubbly, and the toppings are heated through.

10 Once the pizza is cooked to your liking, remove it from the oven and let it cool for a few minutes before slicing. Garnish with fresh basil leaves if desired, then slice and serve.

COOKING TIPS

- Ensure that the cauliflower crust is baked until golden brown before adding the toppings to prevent it from becoming soggy.
- You can customize the pizza toppings according to your preferences. Feel free to add additional vegetables, cooked meats, or your favorite cheeses.
- For a crispier crust, you can flip the cauliflower crust halfway through baking to ensure even cooking on both sides.

HEALTH BENEFITS

- Cauliflower is low in calories and carbohydrates, making it an excellent alternative to traditional pizza crust for those following a low-carb or keto diet.
- Mushrooms are rich in vitamins, minerals, and antioxidants, such as selenium and vitamin D, which may help boost immune function and reduce inflammation.
- Pepperoni provides protein and flavor to the pizza, but opt for leaner varieties or turkey pepperoni to reduce saturated fat and sodium content.

NUTRITIONAL VALUES (PER SERVING):

- **Calories**: 250
- **Total Fat**: 15g
- **Saturated Fat**: 6g
- **Cholesterol**: 60mg
- **Sodium**: 600mg
- **Total Carbohydrates**: 10g
- **Dietary Fiber**: 3g
- **Sugars**: 3g
- **Protein**: 20g

SPICY SHRIMP STIR-FRY WITH CAULIFLOWER RICE RECIPE

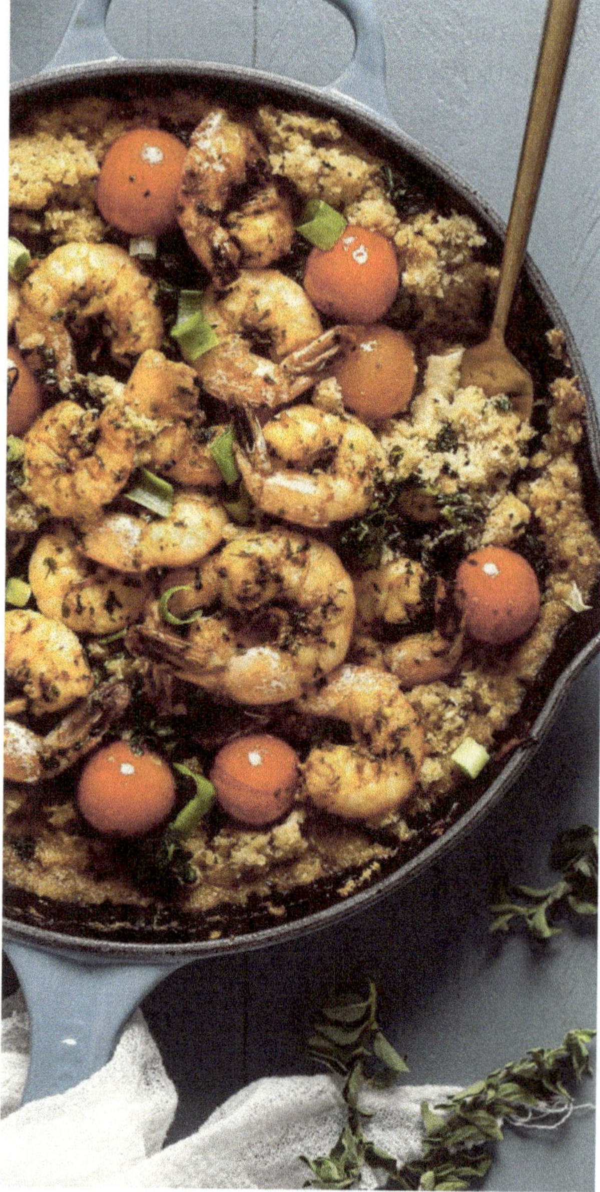

- **Preparation Time:** 15 minutes
- **Cooking Time:** 10 minutes
- **Servings:** 4

INGREDIENTS:

For the spicy shrimp:
- 1 lb (450g) large shrimp, peeled and deveined
- 2 tablespoons soy sauce
- One tablespoon of spicy sauce (to taste)
- 2 cloves garlic, minced
- 1 teaspoon grated fresh ginger
- 1 tablespoon sesame oil
- 1 tablespoon olive oil
- Salt and pepper to taste

For the stir-fry:
- 1 medium head cauliflower, cut into florets
- 1 tablespoon olive oil
- 1 bell pepper, thinly sliced
- 1 cup broccoli florets
- 1/2 cup sliced carrots
- 1/4 cup sliced green onions
- Sesame seeds for garnish (optional)

PROCEDURES:

1. In a bowl, combine the soy sauce, sriracha sauce, minced garlic, grated ginger, sesame oil, olive oil, salt, and pepper. Toss the shrimp in the basin to ensure consistent coating. Let it marinate for 10 minutes.
2. Meanwhile, make the cauliflower rice by pulsing the cauliflower florets in a food processor until they resemble rice grains.
3. In a large skillet or wok, heat 1 tablespoon of olive oil over medium-high heat. When the shrimp are pink and fully cooked, add them to the skillet and sauté them for two to three minutes on each side. After

taking the shrimp out of the skillet, set it aside.

4 In the same skillet, add another tablespoon of olive oil if needed. Add the sliced bell pepper, broccoli florets, and sliced carrots to the skillet. Stir-fry for 3-4 minutes, or until the vegetables are tender-crisp.

5 Add the cauliflower rice to the skillet with the stir-fried vegetables. Cook for an additional 2-3 minutes, stirring frequently, until the cauliflower rice is heated through and slightly tender.

6 Return the cooked shrimp to the skillet with the cauliflower rice and vegetables. Mix everything together until thoroughly hot and properly mixed.

7 Garnish the spicy shrimp stir-fry with sliced green onions and sesame seeds if desired. Serve hot and enjoy!

COOKING TIPS:

- The shrimp can turn rough and rubbery if they are overcooked, so take care not to do that. Just until they become opaque and pink, cook them.
- Adjust the amount of sriracha sauce to your preferred level of spiciness. You can also add red pepper flakes or chili paste for extra heat.
- For added flavor, you can sprinkle the stir-fry with a dash of soy sauce or fish sauce before serving.

- Customize the stir-fry with your favorite vegetables such as snap peas, snow peas, or bok choy.

HEALTH BENEFITS:

- Shrimp is low in calories and fat but high in protein, making it a nutritious option for supporting muscle growth and repair.
- Cauliflower is a low-carb alternative to rice, providing vitamins, minerals, and fiber while helping to keep blood sugar levels stable.
- Bell peppers, broccoli, and carrots are rich in vitamins, minerals, and antioxidants that support overall health and well-being.

NUTRITIONAL VALUES (PER SERVING):

- **Calories**: 250
- **Total Fat**: 12g
- **Saturated Fat**: 2g
- **Cholesterol**: 150mg
- **Sodium**: 600mg
- **Total Carbohydrates**: 10g
- **Dietary Fiber**: 4g
- **Sugars**: 4g
- **Protein**: 25g

GRILLED PORTOBELLO MUSHROOM BURGER WITH AVOCADO RECIPE

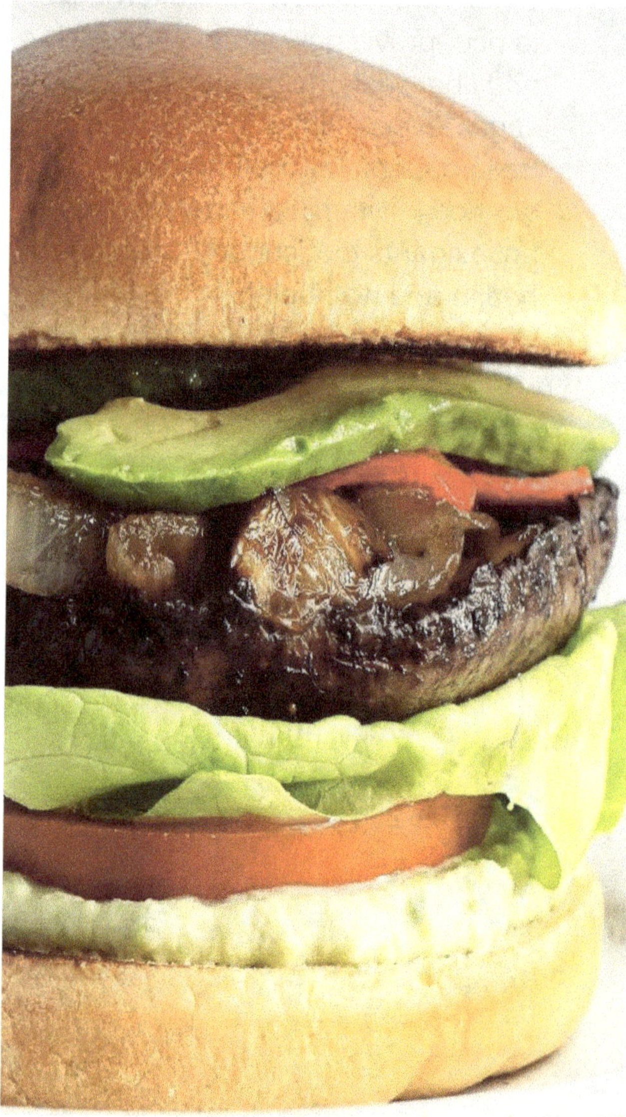

Preparation Time: 15 minutes
Cooking Time: 10 minutes
Servings: 4

INGREDIENTS:

For the grilled portobello mushrooms:

- 4 large portobello mushroom caps
- 2 tablespoons balsamic vinegar
- 2 tablespoons olive oil
- 2 cloves garlic, minced
- Salt and pepper to taste

For assembling the burgers:

- 4 whole grain burger buns
- 1 ripe avocado, sliced
- 1 cup baby spinach leaves
- 1 large tomato, sliced
- 1/4 cup red onion, thinly sliced
- Dijon mustard or your favorite burger sauce

PROCEDURES

1 Clean the portobello mushroom caps by gently wiping them with a damp paper towel to remove any dirt. Remove the stems if necessary.

2 In a shallow dish, whisk together the balsamic vinegar, olive oil, minced garlic, salt, and pepper. Place the mushroom caps in the marinade, turning to coat evenly. Let them marinate for at least 10 minutes, or longer for more flavor.

3 Preheat the grill or grill pan to medium-high heat. Once hot, place the marinated mushroom caps on the grill, gill side down. Grill until soft and gently seared, 4–5 minutes per side.

4 While the mushrooms are grilling, prepare the burger buns and toppings. If preferred, toast the burger buns for one or two minutes on the grill.

5   To assemble the burgers, spread a dollop of Dijon mustard or your favorite burger sauce on the bottom half of each bun. Place a grilled portobello mushroom cap on top, followed by sliced avocado, baby spinach leaves, tomato slices, and thinly sliced red onion.

6   Top each burger with the remaining half of the bun and serve immediately.

COOKING TIPS

- When grilling the portobello mushrooms, be sure to brush off any excess marinade to prevent flare-ups on the grill.
- You can alter the toppings to suit your tastes. Add cheese, pickles, or caramelized onions for extra flavor.
- For a lower-carb option, you can serve the grilled portobello mushrooms without the bun and enjoy them as a hearty salad or side dish.
- If you don't have a grill, you can also cook the portobello mushrooms in a skillet or grill pan on the stovetop.

HEALTH BENEFITS

- Portobello mushrooms are low in calories and fat but rich in fiber, vitamins, and minerals such as potassium and selenium. They also contain antioxidants that may help protect against oxidative stress and inflammation.
- Avocado is a nutrient-dense fruit that provides heart-healthy monounsaturated fats, fiber, and essential vitamins and minerals, including potassium and vitamin K.
- Baby spinach leaves are packed with vitamins A, C, and K, as well as folate, iron, and antioxidants that support immune function and overall health.

NUTRITIONAL VALUES (PER SERVING,

- **Calories**: 300
- **Total Fat**: 15g
- **Saturated Fat**: 2g
- **Cholesterol**: 0mg
- **Sodium**: 300mg
- **Total Carbohydrates**: 35g
- **Dietary Fiber**: 8g
- **Sugars**: 5g
- **Protein**: 10g

NOTE: Nutritional values are approximate and may vary depending on the specific brands and quantities of ingredients used. Adjustments can be made to the recipe to suit individual dietary preferences and requirements.

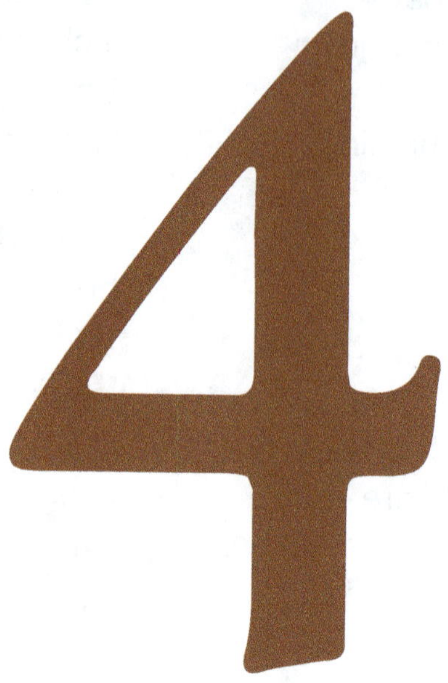

4

SIDE DISHES

GARLIC PARMESAN ROASTED BRUSSELS SPROUTS RECIPE

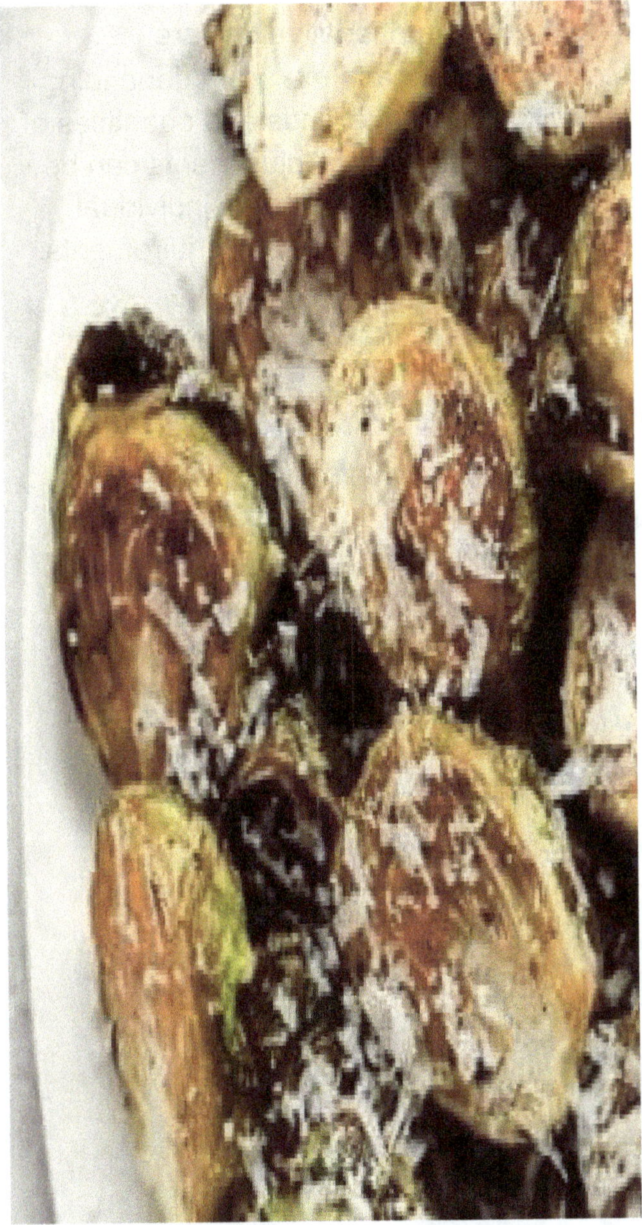

- **Preparation Time**: 10 minutes
- **Cooking Time**: 25 minutes
- **Servings**: 4

INGREDIENTS

- 1 pound (450 grams) of cleaned, halved Brussels sprouts
- 2 tablespoons olive oil
- 2 cloves garlic, minced
- 1/4 cup grated Parmesan cheese
- 1 teaspoon dried thyme
- 1/2 teaspoon garlic powder
- Salt and pepper to taste
- Fresh parsley for garnish (optional)

PROCEDURES

1 Preheat the oven to 400°F (200°C). A baking sheet can be lightly oiled with olive oil or lined with parchment paper.

2 In a large mixing bowl, toss the halved Brussels sprouts with olive oil, minced garlic, grated Parmesan cheese, dried thyme, garlic powder, salt, and pepper until well coated.

3 Spread the seasoned Brussels sprouts in a single layer on the prepared baking sheet, making sure they are evenly spaced to allow for even roasting.

4 Roast the Brussels sprouts in the preheated oven for 20-25 minutes, or until they are tender and golden brown, stirring halfway through cooking to ensure even browning.

5 Once the Brussels sprouts are roasted to perfection, remove them from the oven and transfer them to a serving dish. If preferred, garnish with fresh parsley and serve hot.

COOKING TIPS

- Choose Brussels sprouts that are firm, bright green, and free from yellowing or blemishes for the best flavor and texture.

- Make sure to trim the stem ends of the Brussels sprouts and remove any outer leaves that are damaged or discolored before halving them.
- For extra crispy Brussels sprouts, you can increase the oven temperature to 425°F (220°C) and roast them for a shorter amount of time, checking for doneness after 15-20 minutes.
- To prevent the Brussels sprouts from sticking to the baking sheet, you can toss them with a little extra olive oil or use a silicone baking mat instead of parchment paper.

HEALTH BENEFITS

- Brussels sprouts are rich in vitamins C and K, as well as fiber, antioxidants, and anti-inflammatory compounds that may help support heart health, digestion, and immune function.
- Garlic contains sulfur compounds with potential antibacterial and immune-boosting properties, as well as antioxidants that may help reduce inflammation and lower cholesterol levels.
- Parmesan cheese adds a savory flavor and provides protein, calcium, and phosphorus, which are essential for bone health and muscle function.

NUTRITIONAL VALUES (PER SERVING):

- **Calories**: 150
- **Total Fat**: 10g
- **Saturated Fat**: 2g
- **Cholesterol**: 5mg
- **Sodium**: 200mg
- **Total Carbohydrates**: 10g
- **Dietary Fiber**: 4g
- **Sugars**: 2g
- **Protein**: 6g

NOTE: Nutritional values are approximate and may vary depending on the specific brands and quantities of ingredients used. Adjustments can be made to the recipe to suit individual dietary preferences and requirements.

CREAMY CAULIFLOWER MASH RECIPE

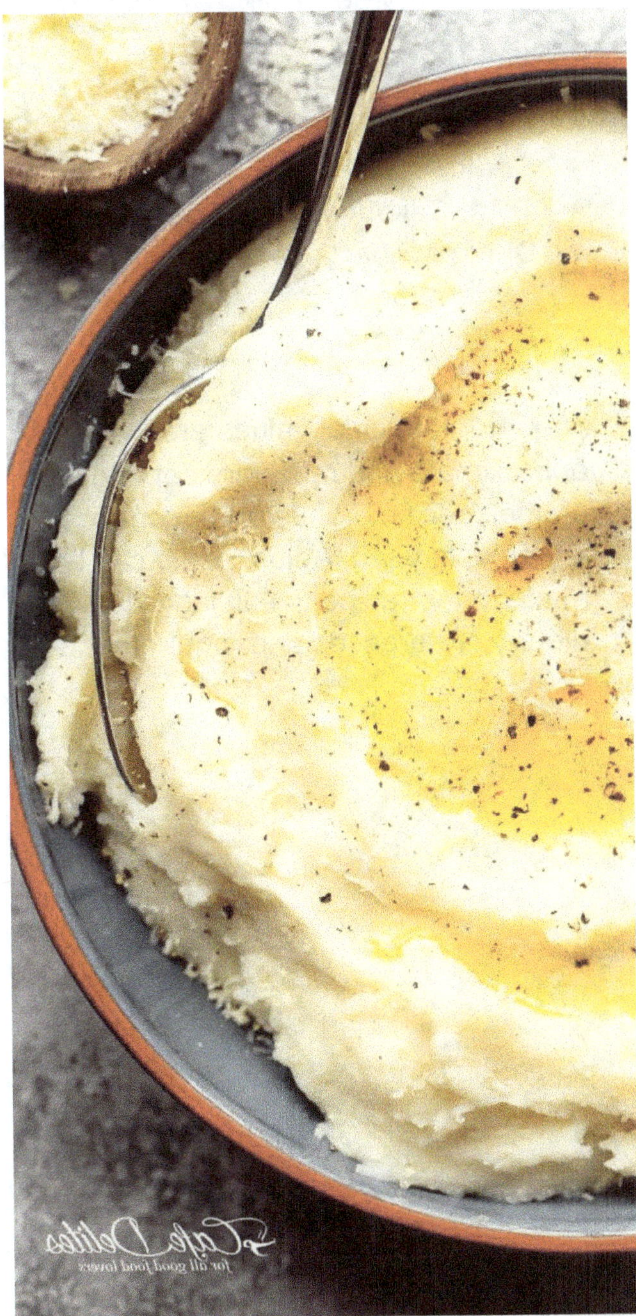

INGREDIENTS:

- 1 large head cauliflower, cut into florets
- 2 cloves garlic, minced
- 2 tablespoons unsalted butter
- 1/4 cup heavy cream
- 1/4 cup grated Parmesan cheese
- Salt and pepper to taste
- Garnish with chopped parsley or chives, if desired.

PROCEDURES

1. Place the cauliflower florets in a large pot and cover with water. Bring the water to a boil over high heat, then reduce the heat to medium-low and simmer for 10-12 minutes, or until the cauliflower is tender when pierced with a fork.
2. While the cauliflower is cooking, melt the butter in a small saucepan over medium heat. When the butter is melted, add the minced garlic and simmer for one to two minutes, or until fragrant.
3. Once the cauliflower is cooked, drain it thoroughly and transfer it to a food processor or blender. Add the garlic butter, heavy cream, grated Parmesan cheese, salt, and pepper to the cauliflower.
4. Blend the cauliflower mixture until smooth and creamy, scraping down the sides of the food processor or blender as needed to ensure even mixing.
5. Taste the creamy cauliflower mash and adjust the seasoning as needed, adding more salt and pepper to taste.

- **Preparation Time**: 10 minutes
- **Cooking Time**: 20 minutes
- **Servings**: 4

6 Transfer the creamy cauliflower mash to a serving bowl and garnish with chopped chives or parsley if desired. Serve hot and enjoy!

COOKING TIPS

- Be sure to drain the cooked cauliflower well before blending to remove excess moisture, as this will help prevent the mash from becoming watery.
- For extra flavor, you can roast the cauliflower florets in the oven before blending. Simply toss them with olive oil, salt, and pepper, and roast at 400°F (200°C) for 20-25 minutes, or until golden brown.
- If you prefer a smoother texture, you can pass the creamy cauliflower mash through a fine-mesh sieve to remove any remaining lumps.
- Feel free to customize the creamy cauliflower mash with your favorite herbs and spices, such as rosemary, thyme, or nutmeg, for added flavor.

HEALTH BENEFITS:

- Cauliflower is low in calories and carbohydrates but rich in vitamins C and K, as well as fiber and antioxidants that support immune function and digestive health.
- Garlic contains sulfur compounds with potential antimicrobial and anti-inflammatory properties, as well as antioxidants that may help reduce the risk of chronic diseases.
- Butter and heavy cream add richness and flavor to the mash while providing essential fats and fat-soluble vitamins such as vitamin A and vitamin E.

NUTRITIONAL VALUES (PER SERVING):

- **Calories**: 150
- **Total Fat**: 12g
- **Saturated Fat**: 8g
- **Cholesterol**: 35mg
- **Sodium**: 150mg
- **Total Carbohydrates**: 8g
- **Dietary Fiber**: 3g
- **Sugars**: 3g
- **Protein**: 4g

NOTE: Nutritional values are approximate and may vary depending on the specific brands and quantities of ingredients used. Adjustments can be made to the recipe to suit individual dietary preferences and requirements.

KETO-FRIENDLY COLESLAW WITH HOMEMADE DRESSING RECIPE

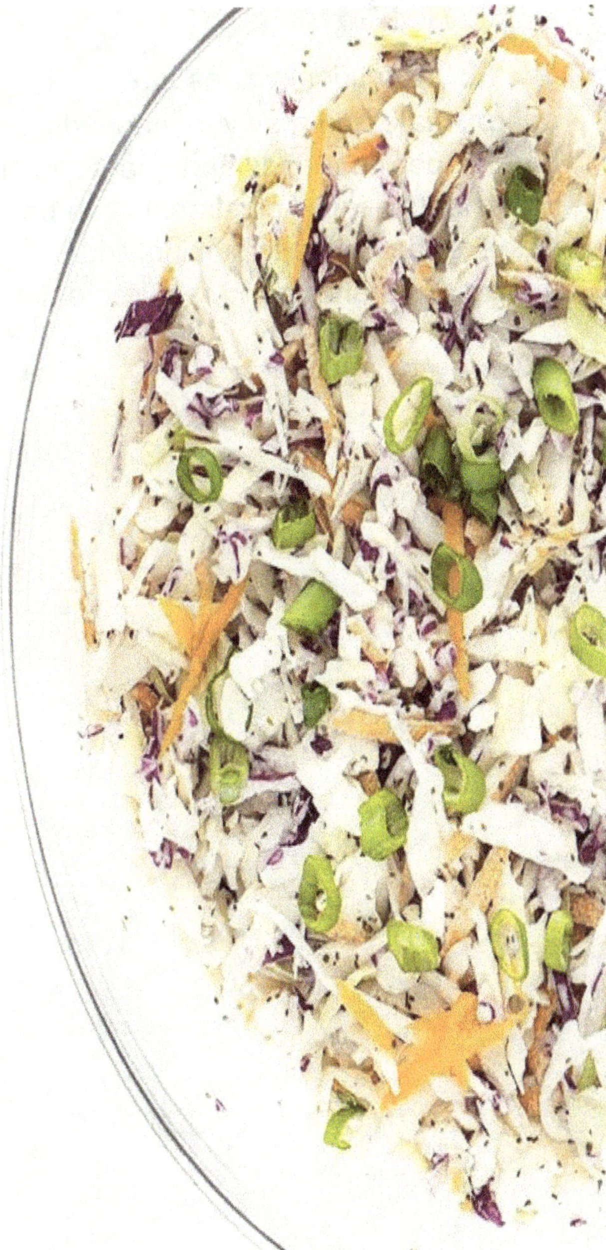

- **Preparation Time**: 15 minutes
- **Servings**: 6

INGREDIENTS

For the coleslaw:

- 1 small head green cabbage, shredded
- 2 medium carrots, grated
- 1/2 small red onion, thinly sliced
- 1/4 cup fresh parsley, chopped

For the dressing:

- 1/2 cup mayonnaise (preferably sugar-free)
- 2 tablespoons apple cider vinegar
- 1 tablespoon Dijon mustard
- 1 teaspoon erythritol or your preferred low-carb sweetener
- 1/2 teaspoon celery seeds
- Salt and pepper to taste

PROCEDURES:

1. Shredded cabbage, grated carrots, finely sliced red onion, and chopped parsley should all be combined in a big mixing dish. Mix the veggies until they are distributed evenly.
2. In a separate bowl, whisk together the mayonnaise, apple cider vinegar, Dijon mustard, erythritol, celery seeds, salt, and pepper to create the coleslaw dressing.
3. Pour the dressing over the cabbage mixture in the large mixing bowl. Use tongs or a large spoon to toss the coleslaw until the vegetables are evenly coated with the dressing.
4. Cover the bowl and refrigerate the coleslaw for at least 30 minutes before serving to allow the flavors to meld together.
5. Once chilled, give the coleslaw a final toss to redistribute the dressing, then serve it as a delicious side dish

or topping for sandwiches, burgers, or tacos.

COOKING TIPS

- For a creamier coleslaw, you can adjust the consistency of the dressing by adding more mayonnaise or a splash of heavy cream.
- To enhance the flavor of the coleslaw, you can add additional ingredients such as chopped green onions, shredded cheese, or crumbled bacon.
- For best results, use a sharp knife or mandoline to thinly slice the cabbage and a box grater or food processor to grate the carrots.

HEALTH BENEFITS

- Cabbage is low in calories and carbohydrates but rich in vitamins C and K, as well as fiber and antioxidants that support immune function and digestive health.
- Carrots are a good source of beta-carotene, which is converted into vitamin A in the body and plays a role in vision health, immune function, and skin health.
- Apple cider vinegar may help improve digestion, regulate blood sugar levels, and promote weight loss when consumed as part of a healthy diet.

NUTRITIONAL VALUES (PER SERVING):

- **Calories**: 150
- **Total Fat**: 12g
- **Saturated Fat**: 2g
- **Cholesterol**: 10mg
- **Sodium**: 200mg
- **Total Carbohydrates**: 6g
- **Dietary Fiber**: 2g
- **Sugars**: 3g
- **Protein**: 1g

NOTE: Nutritional values are approximate and may vary depending on the specific brands and quantities of ingredients used. Adjustments can be made to the recipe to suit individual dietary preferences and requirements.

ROASTED ASPARAGUS WITH LEMON AND PARMESAN RECIPE

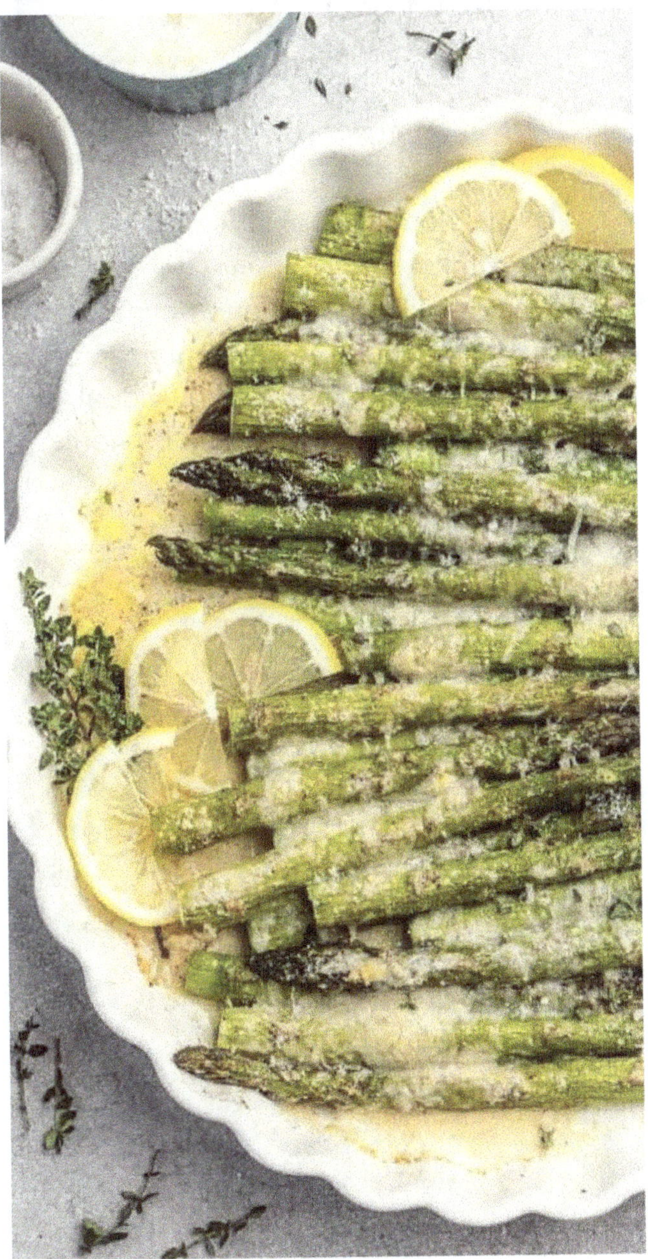

INGREDIENTS:

- 1 lb (450g) asparagus spears, trimmed
- 2 tablespoons olive oil
- 2 cloves garlic, minced
- 1 tablespoon lemon zest
- 2 tablespoons freshly squeezed lemon juice
- 1/4 cup grated Parmesan cheese
- Salt and pepper to taste
- Lemon wedges for serving (optional)

PROCEDURES

1. Preheat the oven to 425°F (220°C). A baking sheet can be lightly oiled with olive oil or lined with parchment paper.
2. Place the trimmed asparagus spears on the prepared baking sheet in a single layer.
3. In a small bowl, whisk together the olive oil, minced garlic, lemon zest, and lemon juice. Drizzle the mixture over the asparagus spears, tossing to coat evenly.
4. Sprinkle the grated Parmesan cheese over the asparagus, then season with salt and pepper to taste.
5. Roast the asparagus in the preheated oven for 10-12 minutes, or until tender and lightly browned, shaking the pan halfway through cooking to ensure even roasting.
6. Once the asparagus is roasted to perfection, remove it from the oven and transfer it to a serving platter. Serve hot, garnished with lemon wedges if desired.

- **Preparation Time:** 10 minutes
- **Cooking Time**: 12 minutes
- **Servings**: 4

COOKING TIPS

- Choose firm, fresh asparagus spears with tightly closed tips and smooth skin for the best flavor and texture.
- To trim the asparagus spears, simply snap off the tough woody ends by bending them near the base. As an alternative, you can cut off the ends with a knife.
- For extra flavor, you can add additional seasonings such as crushed red pepper flakes, dried herbs, or grated garlic to the olive oil mixture before drizzling it over the asparagus.
- Be cautious not to overcook the asparagus, as it can become mushy and lose its vibrant green color. Aim for tender-crisp spears with a slight bite.

HEALTH BENEFITS

- Asparagus is low in calories and carbohydrates but rich in fiber, vitamins A, C, and K, as well as folate and antioxidants that support digestive health, immune function, and heart health.
- Garlic contains sulfur compounds with potential antimicrobial and anti-inflammatory properties, as well as antioxidants that may help reduce the risk of chronic diseases.
- Lemon zest and juice add a burst of citrus flavor and provide vitamin C, which is essential for collagen production, wound healing, and immune function.

NUTRITIONAL VALUES (PER SERVING):

- **Calories**: 80
- **Total Fat**: 6g
- **Saturated Fat**: 1g
- **Cholesterol**: 5mg
- **Sodium**: 100mg
- **Total Carbohydrates**: 5g
- **Dietary Fiber**: 2g
- **Sugars**: 2g
- **Protein**: 4g

NOTE: Nutritional values are approximate and may vary depending on the specific brands and quantities of ingredients used. Adjustments can be made to the recipe to suit individual dietary preferences and requirements.

CHEESY BACON AND CAULIFLOWER RICE RECIPE

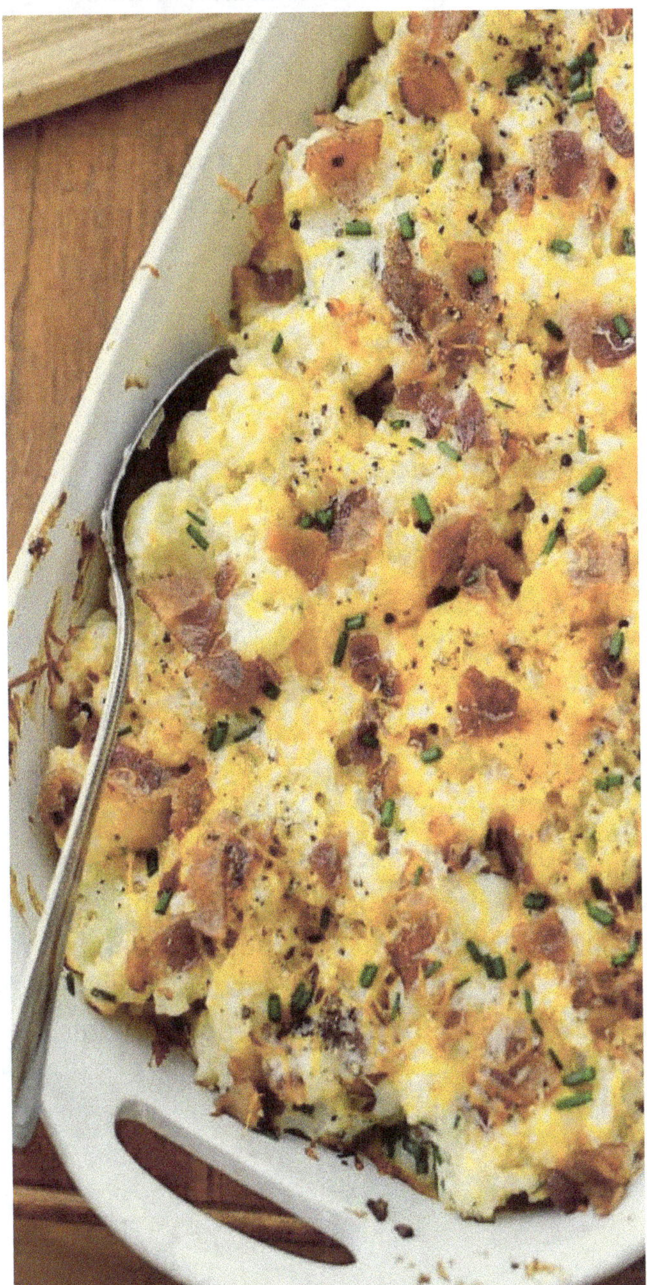

- **Preparation Time**: 10 minutes
- **Cooking Time**: 20 minutes
- **Servings**: 4

INGREDIENTS

- 1 medium head cauliflower, cut into florets
- 4 slices bacon, chopped
- 1 tablespoon butter
- 2 cloves garlic, minced
- 1/2 cup diced onion
- 1 cup shredded cheddar cheese
- Salt and pepper to taste
- Garnish with chopped parsley or chives, if desired.

PROCEDURES:

1 Place the cauliflower florets in a food processor and pulse until they resemble rice grains. As an alternative, you can use a box grater to grind the cauliflower.

2 In a large skillet or frying pan, cook the chopped bacon over medium heat until crispy. Remove the cooked bacon from the pan and drain on paper towels, leaving the bacon fat in the pan.

3 Melt the butter in the skillet containing the bacon fat over a medium flame. Add the minced garlic and diced onion to the skillet, and sauté for 2-3 minutes, or until the onion is translucent and fragrant.

4 Add the riced cauliflower to the skillet with the garlic and onion. Cook for 5-7 minutes, stirring occasionally, until the cauliflower is tender and cooked through.

5 Once the cauliflower is cooked, add the cooked bacon back to the skillet, along with the shredded cheddar cheese. Mix everything together

thoroughly and stir until the cheese has melted.

6   Season the cheesy bacon cauliflower rice with salt and pepper to taste. Garnish with chopped chives or parsley if desired, then serve hot as a delicious side dish or main course.

COOKING TIPS

- Be careful not to overcook the cauliflower rice, as it can become mushy. Cook it just until tender and slightly al dente.
- For added flavor, you can sprinkle the cheesy bacon cauliflower rice with a pinch of smoked paprika or crushed red pepper flakes before serving.
- Customize the recipe with your favorite cheese varieties, such as mozzarella, Monterey Jack, or Gouda, for different flavor profiles.
- You can also add additional vegetables such as diced bell peppers, sliced mushrooms, or chopped spinach to the skillet for extra nutrition and color.

HEALTH BENEFITS

- Cauliflower is low in calories and carbohydrates but rich in fiber, vitamins C and K, as well as antioxidants that support digestive health, immune function, and heart health.
- Bacon adds flavor and protein to the dish, but choose nitrate-free bacon and consume it in moderation to limit saturated fat and sodium intake.
- Cheese provides calcium and protein, but opt for low-fat or reduced-fat varieties to reduce calorie and fat content while still enjoying the cheesy goodness.

NUTRITIONAL VALUES (PER SERVING):

- **Calories**: 250
- **Total Fat**: 18g
- **Saturated Fat**: 10g
- **Cholesterol**: 50mg
- **Sodium**: 400mg
- **Total Carbohydrates**: 8g
- **Dietary Fiber**: 3g
- **Sugars**: 3g
- **Protein**: 14g

NOTE: Nutritional values are approximate and may vary depending on the specific brands and quantities of ingredients used. Adjustments can be made to the recipe to suit individual dietary preferences and requirements.

5

SNACK RECIPES

DR. LESLIE J. STEEN

CHEESE AND PEPPERONI ROLL-UPS RECIPE

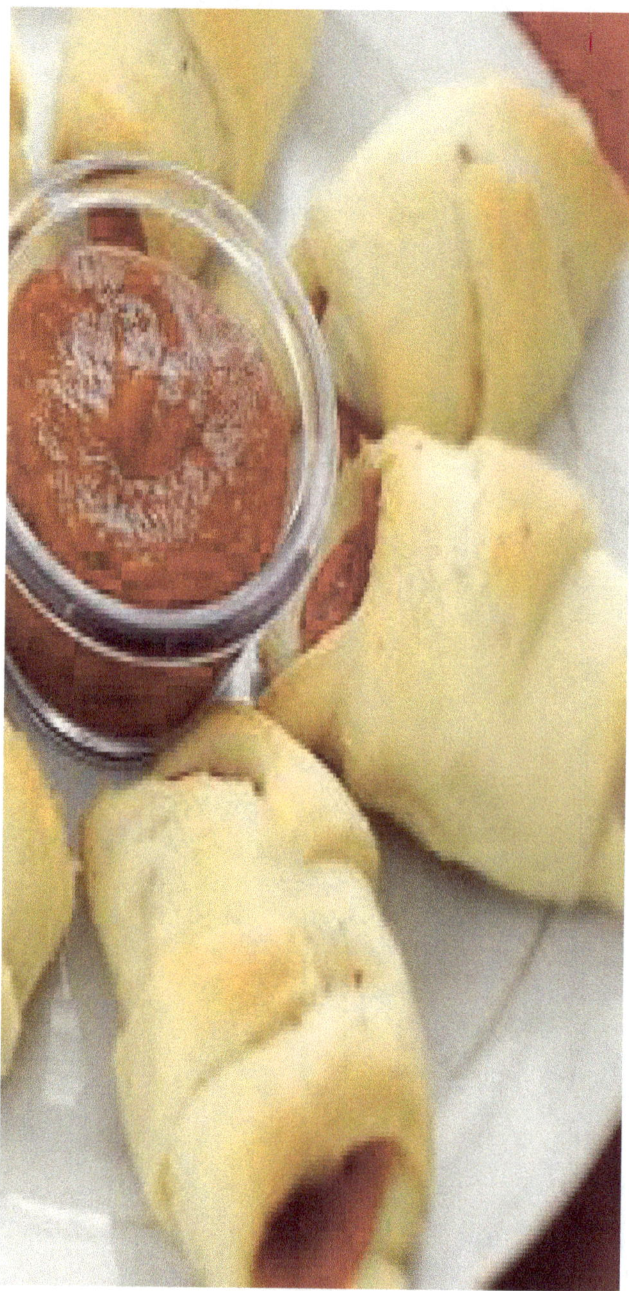

- **Preparation Time**: 10 minutes
- **Cooking Time**: 0 minutes
- **Servings**: 4

INGREDIENTS

- slices pepperoni
- 4 slices mozzarella cheese
- 1/4 cup sliced black olives (optional)
- 1/4 cup sliced cherry tomatoes (optional)
- 1/4 cup sliced bell peppers (optional)
- 1/4 cup sliced cucumber (optional)
- Toothpicks for securing

PROCEDURES

1. Place a slice of mozzarella cheese on a clean surface.
2. Arrange two slices of pepperoni on top of the cheese slice.
3. Add any optional ingredients such as black olives, cherry tomatoes, bell peppers, or cucumber slices on top of the pepperoni.
4. Starting from one end, roll the cheese and pepperoni tightly into a roll-up.
5. Secure the roll-up with a toothpick inserted through the center to hold it in place.
6. Repeat the process with the remaining cheese slices, pepperoni, and optional ingredients to make additional roll-ups.
7. Serve the cheese and pepperoni roll-ups immediately, or store them in an airtight container in the refrigerator for later enjoyment.

COOKING TIPS

- Feel free to customize the roll-ups with your favorite low-carb ingredients such as sliced avocado, pickles, or roasted red peppers for added flavor and variety.

- If you prefer a spicier kick, you can use spicy pepperoni or add a sprinkle of crushed red pepper flakes to the roll-ups before rolling them.
- For a creamier texture, you can spread a thin layer of cream cheese or softened butter on the cheese slices before adding the pepperoni and other toppings.
- Use toothpicks to secure the roll-ups tightly, ensuring that they hold together while being eaten.

HEALTH BENEFITS

- Mozzarella cheese is a good source of protein and calcium, which are essential for muscle and bone health. It also contains vitamin B12 and phosphorus, important for nerve function and energy metabolism.
- Pepperoni provides protein and fats, which help keep you feeling full and satisfied between meals. However, choose nitrate-free pepperoni and consume it in moderation to limit sodium and saturated fat intake.
- Optional vegetables such as black olives, cherry tomatoes, bell peppers, and cucumbers add vitamins, minerals, and fiber to the roll-ups, contributing to overall health and well-being.

NUTRITIONAL VALUES (PER SERVING,

- **Calories**: 120
- **Total Fat**: 10g
- **Saturated Fat**: 5g
- **Cholesterol**: 30mg
- **Sodium**: 250mg
- **Total Carbohydrates**: 2g
- **Dietary Fiber**: 0g
- **Sugars**: 1g
- **Protein**: 8g

NOTE: Nutritional values may vary depending on the specific brands and quantities of ingredients used. Adjustments can be made to the recipe to suit individual dietary preferences and requirements.

GUACAMOLE WITH LOW-CARB VEGGIE STICKS RECIPE

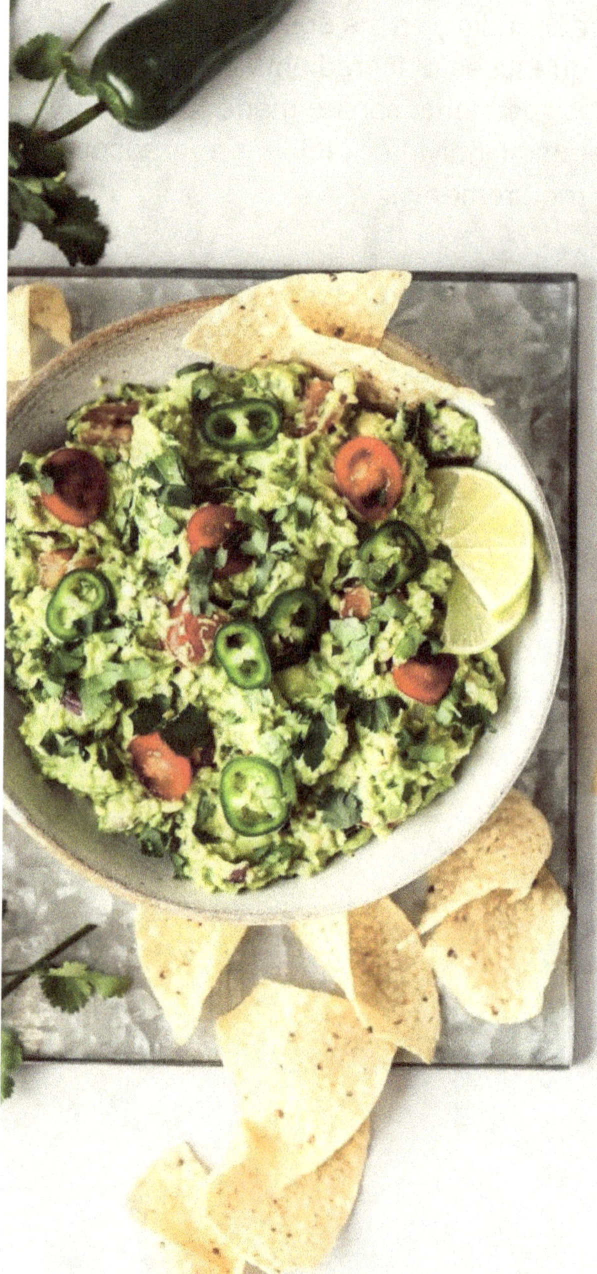

- **Preparation Time**: 10 minutes
- **Cooking Time**: 0 minutes
- **Servings**: 4

INGREDIENTS

For the guacamole:

- 2 ripe avocados
- 1 lime, juiced
- 1/4 cup diced red onion
- 1 small tomato, diced
- 1/4 cup chopped fresh cilantro
- 1 clove garlic, minced
- Salt and pepper to taste

For the low-carb veggie sticks:

- Two medium carrots, sliced into sticks after peeling
- 2 medium cucumbers, cut into sticks
- 2 bell peppers (assorted colors), cut into sticks

PROCEDURES

1. Start by making the guacamole. Remove the pits from the avocados, cut them in half, and scoop the flesh into a mixing bowl.
2. Using a fork, mash the avocados until they are smooth but still have some chunks.
3. Add the lime juice, diced red onion, diced tomato, chopped cilantro, minced garlic, salt, and pepper to the mashed avocados. Stir until well combined.
4. Taste the guacamole and adjust the seasoning as needed, adding more salt, pepper, or lime juice to suit your preferences.
5. Prepare the low-carb veggie sticks by peeling and cutting the carrots into sticks, cutting the cucumbers into sticks, and cutting the bell peppers into sticks.

6   Arrange the veggie sticks on a serving platter alongside the guacamole.

7   Serve the guacamole with the low-carb veggie sticks for dipping, and enjoy!

COOKING TIPS

- To prevent the guacamole from browning, place plastic wrap directly on the surface of the guacamole and refrigerate until ready to serve.
- For added flavor and spice, you can add diced jalapeño peppers or a pinch of cayenne pepper to the guacamole.
- Customize the low-carb veggie sticks with your favorite vegetables such as celery, jicama, or radishes for variety and color.
- To make ahead, prepare the guacamole and store it in an airtight container in the refrigerator for up to 1 day. Cut the vegetables into sticks and store them in separate containers until ready to serve.

HEALTH BENEFITS

- Avocados are loaded with heart-healthy monounsaturated fats, fiber, and vitamins such as vitamin K, vitamin E, and vitamin C. Additionally, potassium is included in them, which aids in controlling blood pressure and fluid balance.
- Tomatoes are rich in lycopene, an antioxidant that may help protect against certain types of cancer and cardiovascular disease. They also supply fiber, potassium, and vitamins A and C.
- Bell peppers are low in calories and carbohydrates but high in vitamins A and C, as well as antioxidants that support eye health, immune function, and skin health.
- Cucumbers are hydrating and low in calories, making them a refreshing and nutritious snack. They also provide vitamins K and C, as well as silica, which promotes healthy skin and joints.

NUTRITIONAL VALUES (PER SERVING, BASED ON BASIC INGREDIENTS):

- **Calories**: 150
- **Total Fat**: 11g
- **Saturated Fat**: 2g
- **Cholesterol**: 0mg
- **Sodium**: 10mg
- **Total Carbohydrates**: 14g
- **Dietary Fiber**: 8g
- **Sugars**: 4g
- **Protein**: 3g

NOTE: Nutritional values may vary depending on the specific brands and quantities of ingredients used. Adjustments can be made to the recipe to suit individual dietary preferences and requirements.

SPICY BUFFALO CAULIFLOWER BITES RECIPE

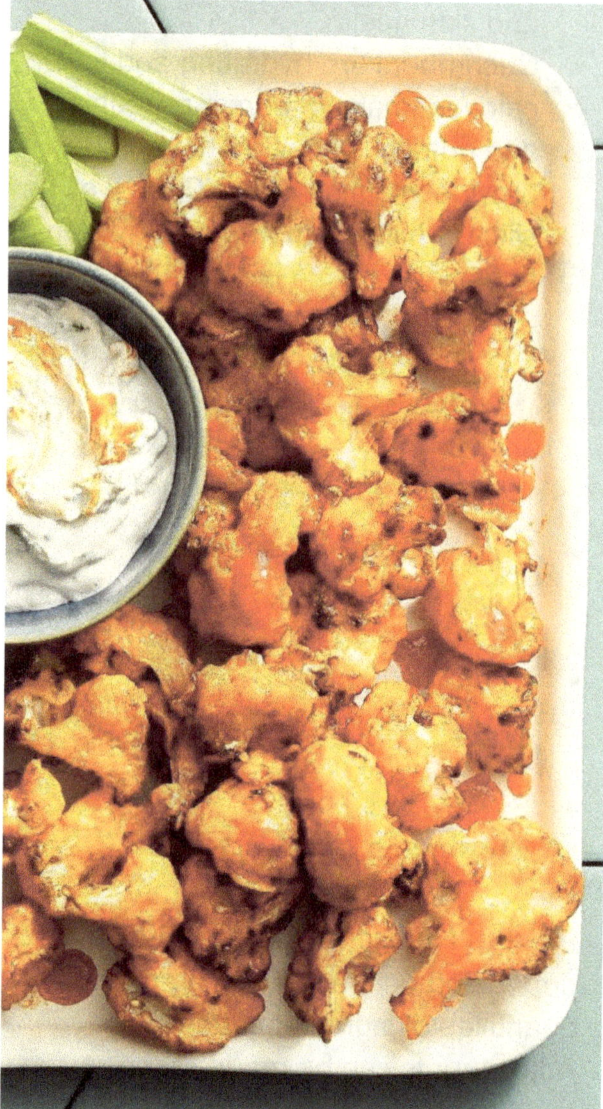

- **Preparation Time:** 15 minutes
- **Cooking Time:** 25 minutes
- **Servings:** 4

INGREDIENTS

For the cauliflower bites:

- 1 head cauliflower, cut into florets
- 1/2 cup almond flour or coconut flour
- 1 teaspoon garlic powder
- 1 teaspoon paprika
- 1/2 teaspoon salt
- 1/4 teaspoon black pepper
- Cooking spray

For the buffalo sauce:

- 1/4 cup hot sauce (such as Frank's RedHot)
- 2 tablespoons unsalted butter, melted
- 1 tablespoon apple cider vinegar
- 1/2 teaspoon Worcestershire sauce
- 1/2 teaspoon garlic powder
- 1/4 teaspoon cayenne pepper (optional, for extra heat)

For serving:

- Ranch or blue cheese dressing
- Celery sticks
- Carrot sticks

PROCEDURES

1. Preheat the oven to 425°F (220°C). Line a baking sheet with parchment paper or lightly grease with cooking spray.
2. In a large mixing bowl, combine the almond flour (or coconut flour), garlic powder, paprika, salt, and black pepper. Mix well to combine.
3. Toss the cauliflower florets in the seasoned flour mixture until evenly coated.
4. Place the coated cauliflower florets in a single layer on the baking sheet that has been prepared.
5. . Make sure they are not touching each other to ensure even crisping.
6. Spray the cauliflower florets lightly with cooking spray to help them brown and crisp up in the oven.

7 Bake the cauliflower bites in the preheated oven for 20-25 minutes, or until they are golden brown and crispy, flipping halfway through cooking to ensure even browning.

8 While the cauliflower is baking, prepare the buffalo sauce. In a small mixing bowl, whisk together the hot sauce, melted butter, apple cider vinegar, Worcestershire sauce, garlic powder, and cayenne pepper (if using) until well combined.

9 Once the cauliflower bites are cooked, transfer them to a large mixing bowl. Pour the buffalo sauce over the cauliflower bites and toss gently to coat evenly.

10 Serve the spicy buffalo cauliflower bites hot with ranch or blue cheese dressing for dipping, along with celery sticks and carrot sticks on the side.

COOKING TIPS

- Make sure to cut the cauliflower florets into similar-sized pieces to ensure even cooking.
- For extra crispy cauliflower bites, you can use a wire rack set on top of the baking sheet to allow air circulation around the florets while baking.
- Adjust the amount of hot sauce and cayenne pepper in the buffalo sauce according to your desired level of spiciness.
- Serve the buffalo cauliflower bites immediately after tossing them in the sauce to maintain their crispiness.

HEALTH BENEFITS

- Cauliflower is low in calories and carbohydrates but rich in fiber, vitamins C and K, as well as antioxidants that support digestive health, immune function, and heart health.
- Hot sauce contains capsaicin, a compound that may help boost metabolism and reduce appetite, leading to potential weight loss benefits.
- Consuming cauliflower instead of traditional buffalo wings reduces calorie and fat intake while still providing a satisfyingly spicy and flavorful snack option.

NUTRITIONAL VALUES (PER SERVING,

- **Calories**: 150
- **Total Fat:** 10g
- **Saturated Fat:** 4g
- **Cholesterol**: 15mg
- **Sodium**: 500mg
- **Total Carbohydrates**: 10g
- **Dietary Fiber**: 4g
- **Sugars**: 2g
- **Protein**: 5g

ALMOND FLOUR CRACKERS WITH CREAM CHEESE AND SMOKED SALMON RECIPE

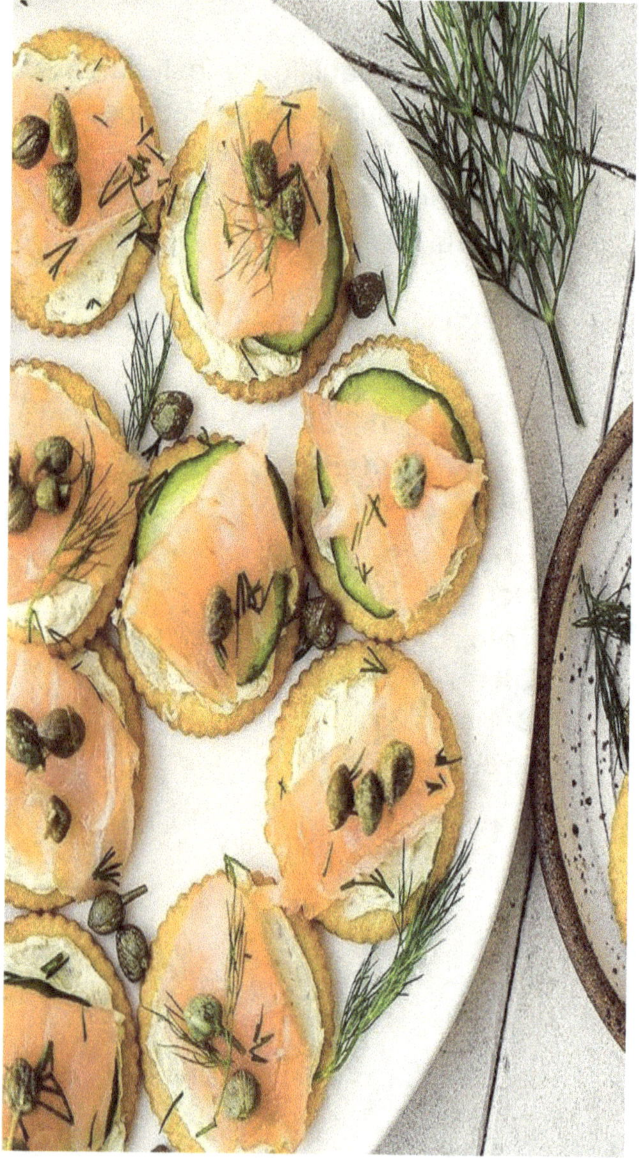

- **Preparation Time**: 20 minutes
- **Cooking Time**: 12-15 minutes
- **Servings**: 4

INGREDIENTS

For the almond flour crackers:

- 1 1/2 cups almond flour
- 1 large egg
- 1 tablespoon olive oil
- 1/2 teaspoon garlic powder
- 1/2 teaspoon onion powder
- 1/4 teaspoon sea salt
- 1/4 teaspoon black pepper
- Sesame seeds, for garnish (optional)

For the toppings:

- 4 ounces cream cheese, softened
- 4 ounces smoked salmon, thinly sliced
- Fresh dill, for garnish (optional)
- Lemon wedges, for serving (optional)

PROCEDURES

1 Preheat the oven to 350°F (175°C). Use parchment paper to line a baking sheet.

2 In a mixing bowl, combine the almond flour, egg, olive oil, garlic powder, onion powder, sea salt, and black pepper. Mix well until a dough forms.

3 Place the dough between two sheets of parchment paper and roll it out thinly, about 1/8 inch thick.

4 Use a knife or pizza cutter to cut the rolled-out dough into small squares or rectangles to form crackers. Optionally, you can use a cookie cutter to create various shapes.

5 Transfer the cut crackers to the prepared baking sheet, leaving some space between each cracker.

6   If desired, sprinkle sesame seeds over the crackers for added flavor and texture.

7   Bake the crackers in the preheated oven for 12-15 minutes, or until golden brown and crispy. Keep an eye on them as almond flour can burn quickly.

8   Once baked, remove the crackers from the oven and let them cool completely on the baking sheet.

9   To assemble, spread a layer of softened cream cheese on each almond flour cracker.

10   Top each cracker with a slice of smoked salmon.

11   Garnish with fresh dill, if desired, and serve with lemon wedges on the side for squeezing over the smoked salmon.

COOKING TIPS

- Make sure to roll out the dough thinly to achieve crispy crackers. If the dough is too thick, the crackers may be chewy instead of crispy.
- You can customize the flavor of the almond flour crackers by adding herbs or spices to the dough, such as rosemary, thyme, or chili flakes.
- For an extra burst of flavor, you can sprinkle the crackers with everything bagel seasoning before baking.
- Store any leftover almond flour crackers in an airtight container at room temperature for up to 3 days. They can be frozen as well for extended storage.

HEALTH BENEFITS

- Almond flour is low in carbs and high in healthy fats, fiber, and protein, making it a nutritious alternative to traditional wheat flour.
- Omega-3 fatty acids, which are good for the heart, brain, and body's ability to reduce inflammation.
- Cream cheese provides calcium, protein, and fat, which help keep youfeeling full and satisfied.

NUTRITIONAL VALUES (PER SERVING, BASED ON BASIC INGREDIENTS):

- **Calories**: 300
- **Total Fat**: 24g
- **Saturated Fat**: 6g
- **Cholesterol**: 65mg
- **Sodium**: 450mg
- **Total Carbohydrates**: 10g
- **Dietary Fiber**: 4g
- **Sugars**: 2g
- **Protein**: 14g

CUCUMBER AVOCADO SALSA RECIPE

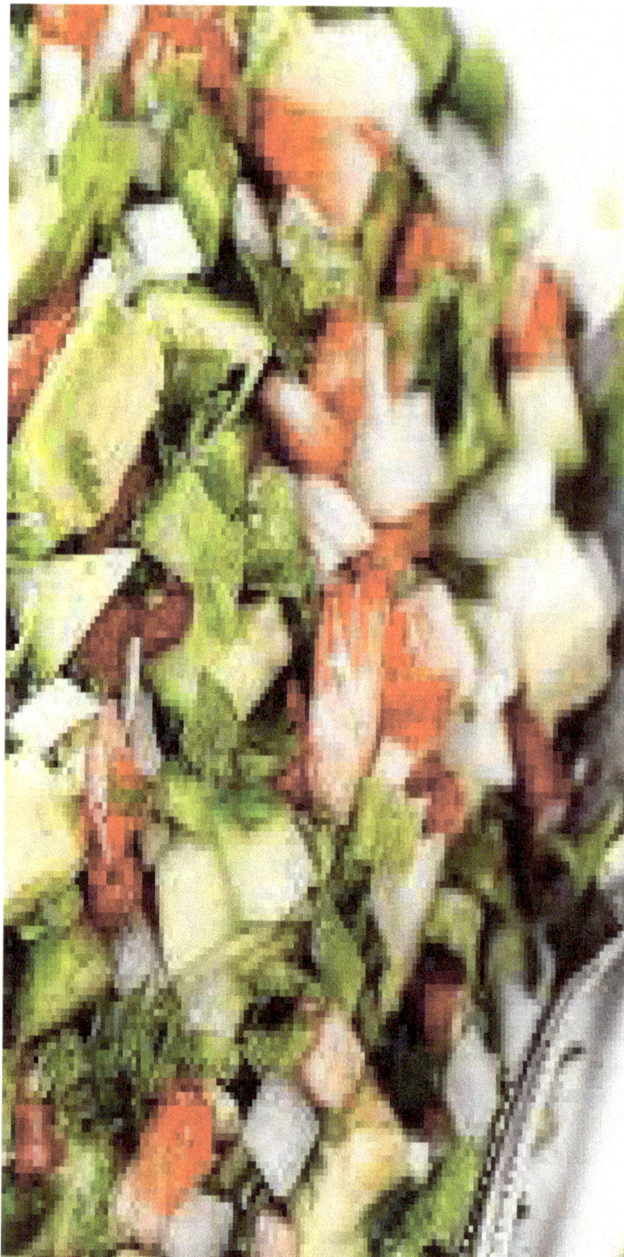

- **Preparation Time**: 15 minutes
- **Cooking Time**: 0 minutes
- **Servings**: 4

INGREDIENTS

- 1 large cucumber, diced
- 1 ripe avocado, diced
- 1/2 cup cherry tomatoes, halved
- 1/4 cup red onion, finely chopped
- 1/4 cup fresh cilantro, chopped
- 1 minced and seeded jalapeño pepper (optional)
- 1 lime, juiced
- 1 tablespoon extra virgin olive oil
- Salt and pepper to taste

PROCEDURES

1. In a large mixing bowl, combine the diced cucumber, diced avocado, halved cherry tomatoes, finely chopped red onion, chopped cilantro, and minced jalapeño pepper (if using).
2. Drizzle the lime juice and extra virgin olive oil over the ingredients in the bowl.
3. Gently toss the ingredients together until well combined, ensuring that the avocado pieces are evenly coated with the lime juice to prevent browning.
4. Season the cucumber avocado salsa with salt and pepper to taste, adjusting the seasoning as needed.
5. Allow the flavors to meld together by refrigerating the salsa for at least 15 minutes before serving.
6. Once chilled, give the salsa a final stir, then serve it as a refreshing and flavorful topping for grilled meats, fish, tacos, or as a dip with tortilla chips.

COOKING TIPS:

- Choose a ripe avocado that yields slightly to gentle pressure when squeezed, but is not overly soft or mushy.
- If you prefer a milder salsa, you can omit the jalapeño pepper or remove the seeds and membranes before mincing to reduce the heat level.
- For extra flavor, you can add additional ingredients such as diced mango, pineapple, or black beans to the salsa for sweetness and texture variation.
- To save time, you can use a pre-made salsa verde or pico de gallo as a base and simply add diced cucumber and avocado to customize it to your liking.

HEALTH BENEFITS:

- Cucumber is low in calories and carbohydrates but high in water content, making it hydrating and refreshing. It also provides vitamins K and C, as well as antioxidants that support hydration, digestion, and skin health.
- Avocado is a nutrient-dense fruit that is rich in heart-healthy monounsaturated fats, fiber, vitamins E, K, and B6, as well as potassium, which helps regulate blood pressure and fluid balance.
- Tomatoes are a good source of vitamins A, C, and K, as well as antioxidants such as lycopene, which may help reduce the risk of certain types of cancer and cardiovascular disease.

NUTRITIONAL VALUES (PER SERVING, BASED ON BASIC INGREDIENTS):

- **Calories**: 120
- **Total Fat**: 10g
- **Saturated** Fat: 1.5g
- **Cholesterol**: 0mg
- **Sodium**: 10mg
- **Total Carbohydrates**: 8g
- **Dietary Fiber**: 4g
- **Sugars**: 2g
- **Protein**: 2g

NOTE: Nutritional values may vary depending on the specific brands and quantities of ingredients used. Adjustments can be made to the recipe to suit individual dietary preferences and requirements.

6

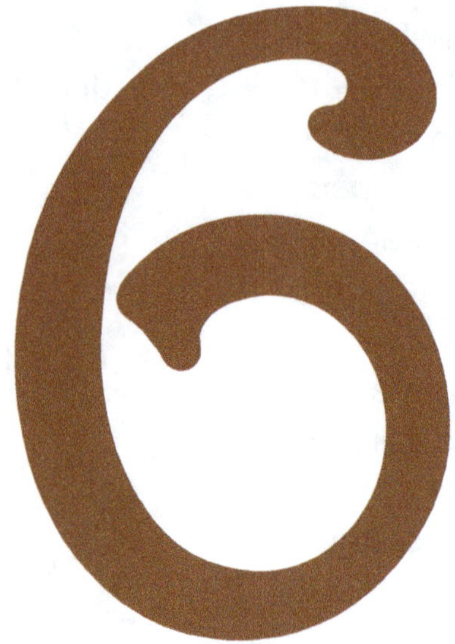

DESSERT RECIPES

DR. LESLIE J. STEEN

KETO CHOCOLATE AVOCADO PUDDING RECIPE

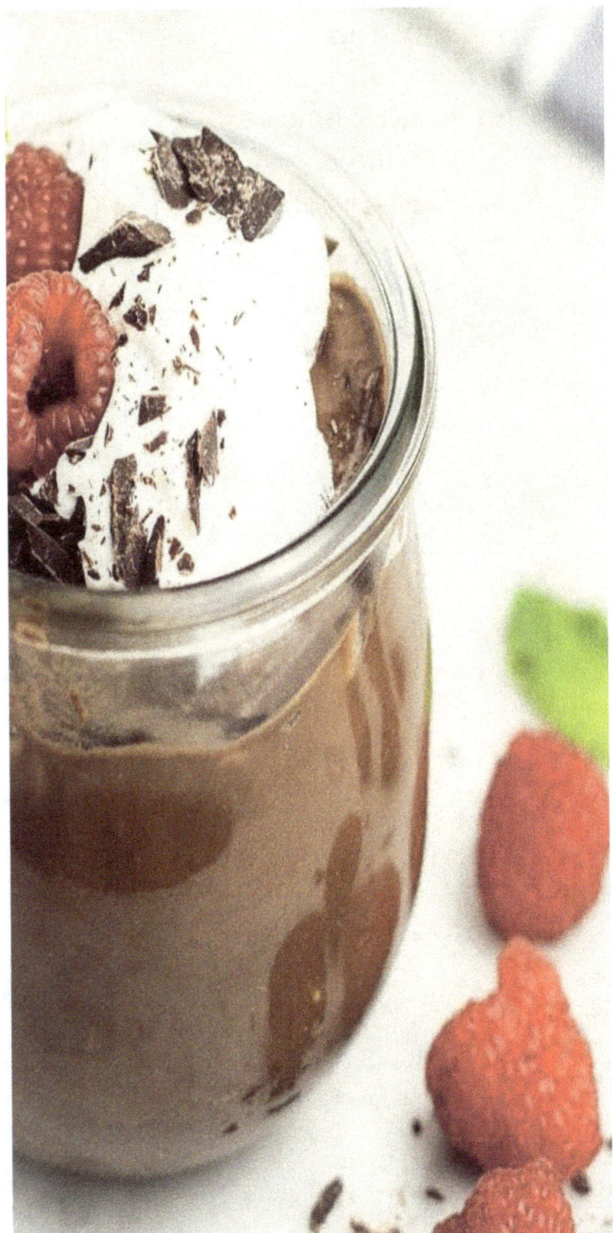

- **Preparation Time**: 10 minutes
- **Cooking Time**: 0 minutes
- **Servings**: 4

INGREDIENTS

- 2 ripe avocados
- 1/4 cup unsweetened cocoa powder
- 1/4 cup almond milk (or any low-carb milk of your choice)
- 1/4 cup powdered erythritol (or sweetener of your choice, to taste)
- 1 teaspoon vanilla extract
- Pinch of salt
- As a garnish, add optional whipped cream and shaved dark chocolate.

PROCEDURES

1. Halve the avocados, remove the pits, and transfer the flesh to a food processor or blender.
2. Add the unsweetened cocoa powder, almond milk, powdered erythritol, vanilla extract, and a pinch of salt to the blender or food processor.
3. Blend the ingredients until smooth and creamy, scraping down the sides of the blender or food processor as needed to ensure everything is well combined.
4. Taste the pudding and adjust the sweetness or cocoa powder to your liking, adding more sweetener if desired for a sweeter taste or more cocoa powder for a richer chocolate flavor.
5. Once the pudding reaches your desired consistency and taste, transfer it to serving bowls or glasses.
6. Chill the pudding in the refrigerator for at least 30 minutes to allow it to set and thicken slightly.
7. Before serving, garnish the chocolate avocado pudding with a

dollop of whipped cream and shaved dark chocolate, if desired.

8 Serve the pudding chilled and enjoy its rich, creamy texture and indulgent chocolate flavor.

COOKING TIPS

- Make sure to use ripe avocados for the creamiest texture and best flavor in the pudding.
- To suit your tastes, adjust the amount of sweetener. You can use powdered erythritol, stevia, monk fruit sweetener, or any other keto-friendly sweetener of your choice.
- For a smoother pudding, you can strain the mixture through a fine-mesh sieve after blending to remove any remaining avocado fibers.
- To make the pudding extra decadent, you can add a tablespoon of unsweetened almond butter or coconut cream to the mixture before blending.

HEALTH BENEFITS

- Avocados are rich in heart-healthy monounsaturated fats, fiber, vitamins E, K, and B6, as well as potassium, which helps regulate blood pressure and fluid balance.
- Unsweetened cocoa powder is a good source of antioxidants, particularly flavonoids, which have been linked to various health benefits, including improved heart health, reduced inflammation, and enhanced cognitive function.
- Almond milk is low in calories and carbohydrates and contains no lactose, making it suitable for those with lactose intolerance or following a dairy-free diet.

NUTRITIONAL VALUES (PER SERVING):

- **Calories**: 180
- **Total Fat**: 15g
- **Saturated Fat**: 2g
- **Cholesterol**: 0mg
- **Sodium**: 10mg
- **Total Carbohydrates**: 11g
- **Dietary Fiber**: 8g
- **Sugars**: 1g
- **Protein**: 3g

LEMON COCONUT FAT BOMBS RECIPE

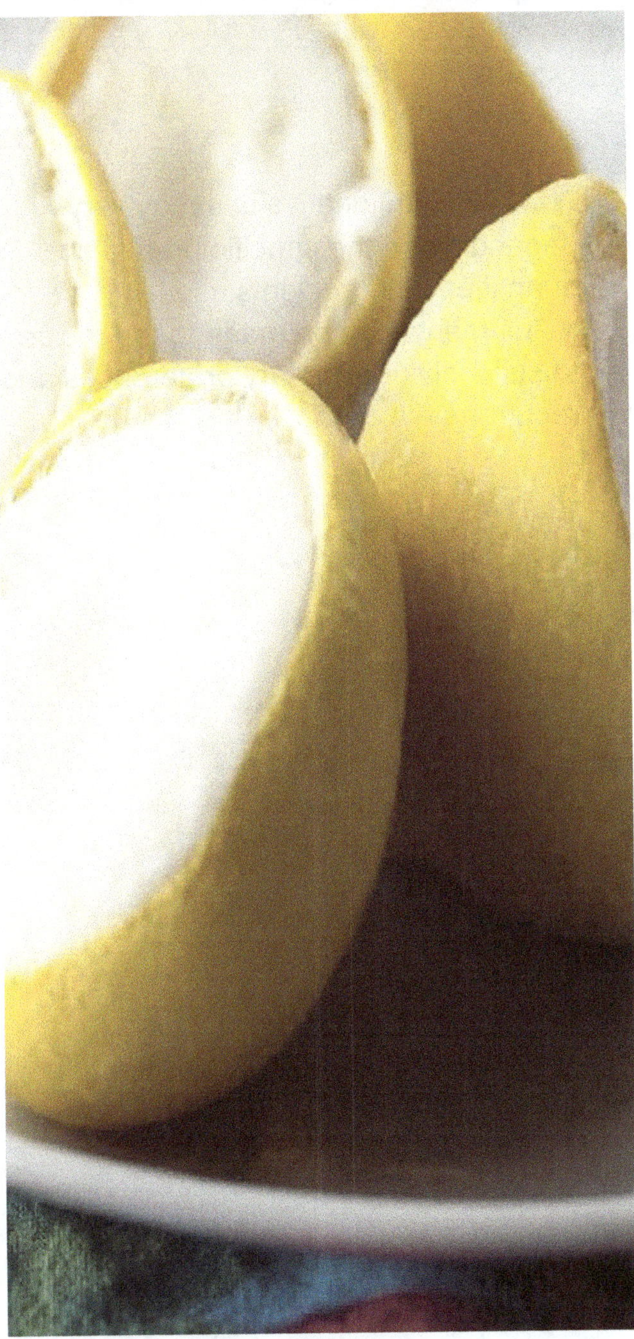

Preparation Time: 15 minutes
Cooking Time: 0 minutes
Chilling Time: 2 hours
Servings: 12 fat bombs

INGREDIENTS

- 1/2 cup coconut oil, melted
- 1/4 cup unsweetened shredded coconut
- Zest of 1 lemon
- 2 tablespoons lemon juice
- 2 tablespoons powdered erythritol (or sweetener of choice)
- 1/2 teaspoon vanilla extract
- Pinch of salt

PROCEDURES

1. In a mixing bowl, combine the melted coconut oil, unsweetened shredded coconut, lemon zest, lemon juice, powdered erythritol, vanilla extract, and a pinch of salt. Until all components are well incorporated, mix well.
2. Taste the mixture and adjust the sweetness or lemon flavor to your liking by adding more powdered erythritol or lemon juice if desired.
3. Once the mixture is well combined and flavored to your preference, spoon it into silicone molds or mini muffin liners, filling each mold or liner about halfway full.
4. Smooth the tops of the fat bombs with a spatula or the back of a spoon to ensure they are level.
5. Place the filled molds or liners in the refrigerator and chill the fat bombs for at least 2 hours, or until they are firm and set.
6. Once the fat bombs are chilled and firm, remove them from the molds or liners and transfer them to an airtight container for storage.

7. Store the lemon coconut fat bombs in the refrigerator until ready to enjoy.

COOKING TIPS

- Use refined coconut oil if you prefer a more neutral coconut flavor, or virgin coconut oil for a stronger coconut taste.
- To add a pop of color and flavor, you can sprinkle additional lemon zest or shredded coconut on top of the fat bombs before chilling them in the refrigerator.
- If you don't have silicone molds or mini muffin liners, you can also pour the mixture into an ice cube tray to create individual fat bombs.

HEALTH BENEFITS

- Coconut oil is rich in medium-chain triglycerides (MCTs), a type of fat that is easily absorbed and converted into energy by the body. MCTs have been linked to various health benefits, including improved metabolism, weight management, and cognitive function.
- Lemons are a good source of vitamin C, antioxidants, and flavonoids, which have anti-inflammatory and immune-boosting properties. They also add a refreshing citrus flavor to the fat bombs without adding significant calories or carbohydrates.

NUTRITIONAL VALUES (PER FAT BOMB):

- **Calories**: 80
- **Total Fat**: 9g
- **Saturated Fat**: 8g
- **Cholesterol**: 0mg
- **Sodium**: 0mg
- **Total Carbohydrates**: 1g
- **Dietary Fiber**: 0g
- **Sugars**: 0g
- **Protein**: 0g

NOTE: Nutritional values may vary depending on the specific brands and quantities of ingredients used. Adjustments can be made to the recipe to suit individual dietary preferences and requirements.

BERRIES AND CREAM PARFAIT RECIPE

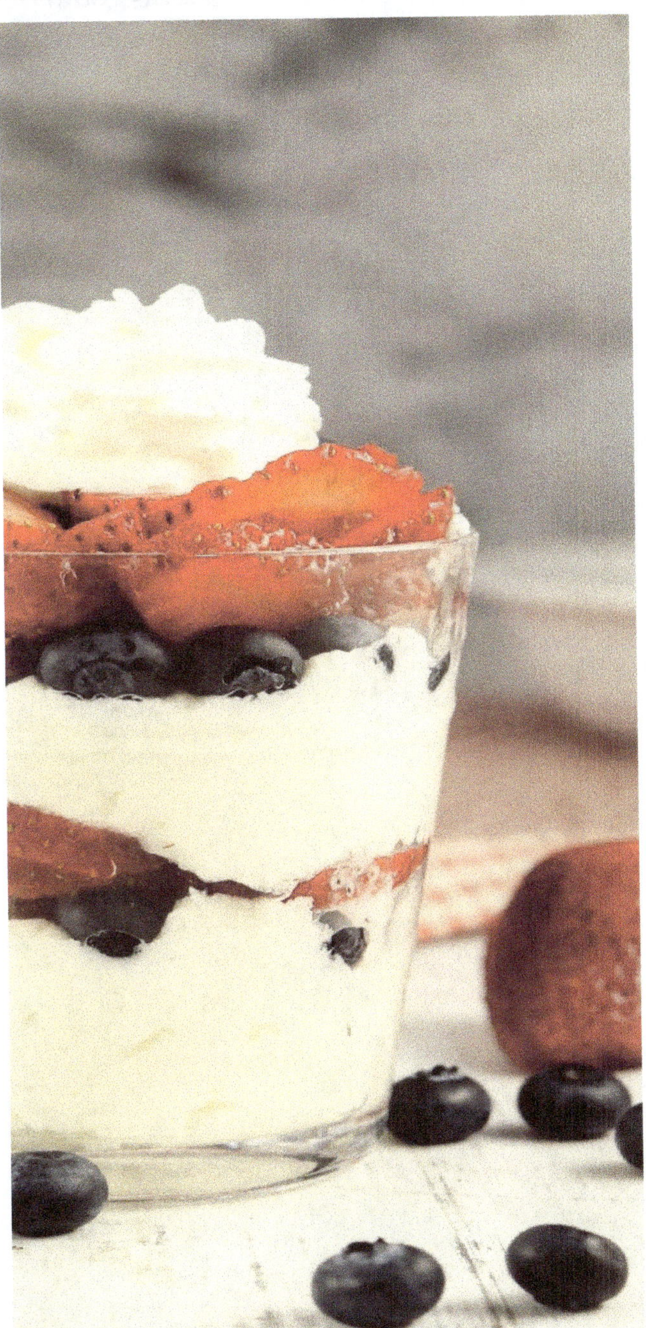

- **Preparation Time**: 15 minutes
- **Cooking Time**: 0 minutes
- **Servings**: 4

INGREDIENTS:

For the parfait layers:

- Two cups of mixed berries, including blueberries, raspberries, strawberries, and blackberries
- One tablespoon of powdered erythritol, or your preferred sweetener
- 1 teaspoon lemon juice
- 1 cup whipped cream or coconut cream

For the optional toppings:

- Fresh mint leaves for garnish
- Unsweetened shredded coconut for sprinkling
- Chopped nuts (such as almonds or walnuts) for crunch

PROCEDURES

- Start by preparing the berries. Wash the mixed berries under cold water and pat them dry with a paper towel. Remove any stems or hulls from the strawberries and slice them into bite-sized pieces if desired.
- In a mixing bowl, combine the mixed berries with the powdered erythritol and lemon juice. Gently toss the berries until they are evenly coated with the sweetener and lemon juice.
- Next, prepare the whipped cream or coconut cream. If using store-bought whipped cream, simply transfer it to a mixing bowl. If making homemade whipped cream, whip chilled heavy cream or coconut cream using a hand mixer or stand mixer until stiff peaks form.

- To assemble the parfaits, begin by layering a spoonful of whipped cream or coconut cream into the bottom of each serving glass or bowl.
- Add a layer of the sweetened mixed berries on top of the whipped cream.
- Repeat the layers, alternating between whipped cream and mixed berries until the glasses or bowls are filled to the desired height.
- Finish the parfaits with a dollop of whipped cream on top and garnish with fresh mint leaves, shredded coconut, and chopped nuts if desired.
- Serve the berries and cream parfaits immediately, or refrigerate them until ready to serve.

COOKING TIPS

- For added flavor, you can sprinkle each layer of whipped cream with a pinch of vanilla bean powder or extract.
- If you prefer a sweeter parfait, you can drizzle each layer of whipped cream with a little honey or maple syrup.
- Customize the parfaits by using your favorite combination of berries or adding other fruits such as sliced peaches, kiwi, or mango.
- To make the parfaits ahead of time, prepare the components separately and assemble them just before serving to prevent the layers from becoming soggy.

HEALTH BENEFITS

- Berries are rich in antioxidants, vitamins, and fiber, which help support overall health and reduce the risk of chronic diseases such as heart disease and cancer.
- Whipped cream or coconut cream adds a creamy texture and satisfying richness to the parfaits while providing healthy fats and a source of energy.

NUTRITIONAL VALUES (PER SERVING):

- **Calories**: 150
- **Total Fat:** 10g
- **Saturated Fat**: 8g
- **Cholesterol**: 0mg
- **Sodium**: 10mg
- **Total Carbohydrates**: 15g
- **Dietary Fiber**: 5g
- **Sugars**: 8g
- **Protein**: 2g

PEANUT BUTTER CHOCOLATE CHIP COOKIES (SUGAR-FREE) RECIPE

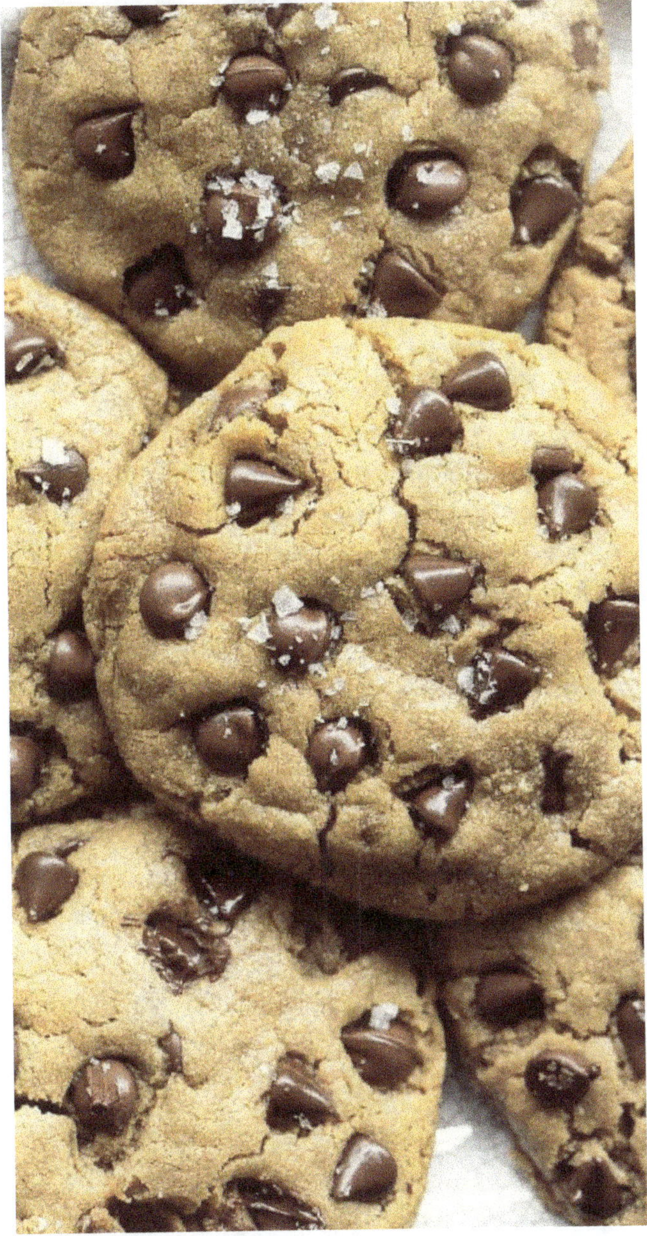

- **Preparation Time**: 15 minutes
- **Cooking Time**: 10-12 minutes
- **Servings**: 12 cookies

INGREDIENTS

- 1 cup natural peanut butter (unsweetened)
- 1/2 cup powdered erythritol (or sweetener of choice)
- 1 large egg
- 1 teaspoon vanilla extract
- 1/4 teaspoon salt
- 1/2 cup sugar-free chocolate chips

PROCEDURES

1. Preheat the oven to 350°F (175°C). Use silicone baking mats or parchment paper to line a baking pan.
2. In a mixing bowl, combine the natural peanut butter, powdered erythritol, egg, vanilla extract, and salt. Mix well until all ingredients are thoroughly combined and a dough forms.
3. Once the sugar-free chocolate chips are well mixed into the cookie batter, fold them in.
4. Using a cookie scoop or spoon, portion out the cookie dough and roll it into balls. The cookie dough balls should be spaced about 2 inches apart on the baking sheet that has been prepared.
5. Use a fork to flatten each cookie dough ball slightly, creating a crisscross pattern on top.
6. Bake the cookies in the preheated oven for 10-12 minutes, or until the edges are golden brown and the cookies are set.
7. Remove the cookies from the oven and let them cool on the baking

sheet for a few minutes before transferring them to a wire rack to cool completely.

8. Once cooled, store the peanut butter chocolate chip cookies in an airtight container at room temperature for up to 5 days.

COOKING TIPS

- Use natural peanut butter without added sugar or oil for the best texture and flavor in the cookies.
- If the cookie dough is too sticky to handle, refrigerate it for 30 minutes to firm it up before shaping the dough into balls.
- For extra flavor and texture, you can add chopped nuts such as almonds, pecans, or walnuts to the cookie dough along with the chocolate chips.
- Be careful not to overbake the cookies, as they can become dry and crumbly. They will continue to firm up as they cool on the baking sheet.

HEALTH BENEFITS

- Peanut butter is a good source of protein, healthy fats, and fiber, which help keep you feeling full and satisfied. It also provides essential nutrients such as vitamin E, magnesium, and potassium.
- Erythritol is a sugar alcohol that provides sweetness without the calories or blood sugar spike associated with regular sugar. It is also tooth-friendly and does not promote tooth decay.

- Sugar-free chocolate chips provide the rich, indulgent flavor of chocolate without the added sugars, making them suitable for those following a low-carb or keto diet.

NUTRITIONAL VALUES (PER SERVING,

- **Calories**: 150
- **Total Fat**: 12g
- **Saturated Fat**: 2g
- **Cholesterol**: 15mg
- **Sodium**: 100mg
- **Total Carbohydrates**: 8g
- **Dietary Fiber**: 2g
- **Sugars**: 1g
- **Protein**: 6g

NOTE: Nutritional values may vary depending on the specific brands and quantities of ingredients used. Adjustments can be made to the recipe to suit individual dietary preferences and requirements.

VANILLA ALMOND BUTTER FAT BOMBS RECIPE

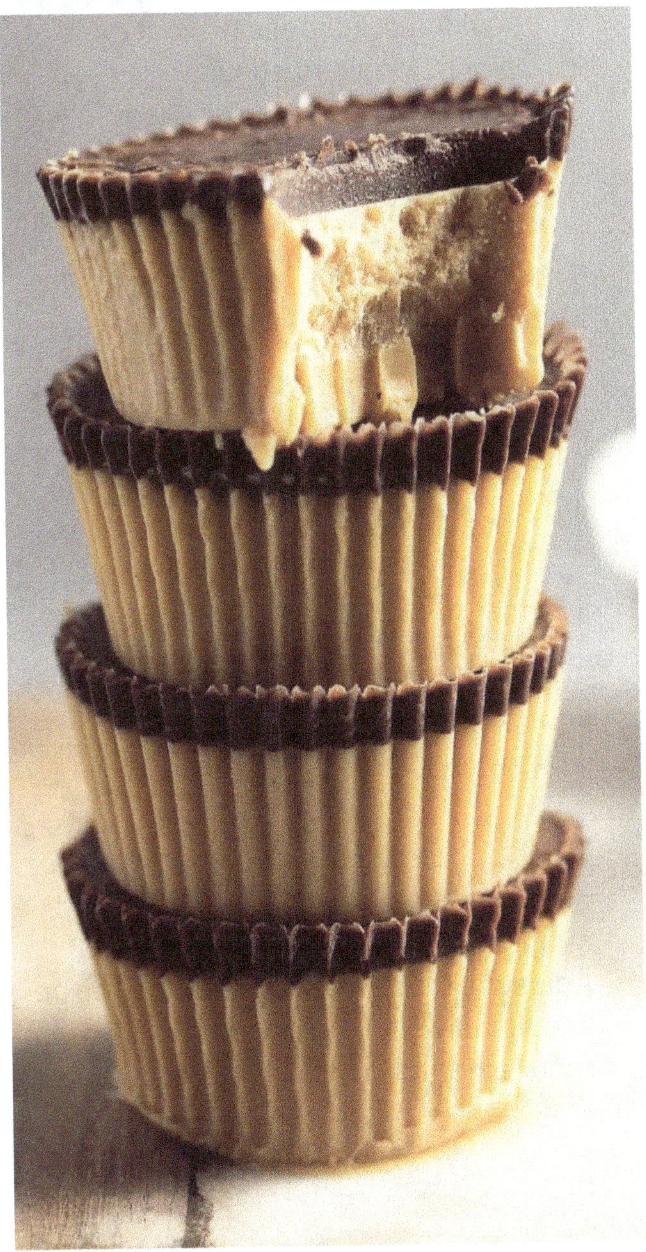

- **Preparation Time**: 10 minutes
- **Cooking Time**: 0 minutes
- **Chilling Time**: 2 hours
- **Servings**: 12 fat bombs

INGREDIENTS

- 1/2 cup almond butter (unsweetened)
- 1/4 cup coconut oil, melted
- 2 tablespoons powdered erythritol (or sweetener of choice)
- 1 teaspoon vanilla extract
- Pinch of salt
- Sliced almonds for garnish (optional)

PROCEDURES

- In a mixing bowl, combine the almond butter, melted coconut oil, powdered erythritol, vanilla extract, and a pinch of salt. Mix well until all ingredients are thoroughly combined and the mixture is smooth.
- Taste the mixture and adjust the sweetness or vanilla flavor to your liking by adding more powdered erythritol or vanilla extract if desired.
- Once the mixture is well combined and flavored to your preference, spoon it into silicone molds or mini muffin liners, filling each mold or liner about halfway full.
- Smooth the tops of the fat bombs with a spatula or the back of a spoon to ensure they are level.
- If desired, garnish each fat bomb with a few sliced almonds for added texture and visual appeal.
- Place the filled molds or liners in the refrigerator and chill the fat bombs for at least 2 hours, or until they are firm and set.
- Once the fat bombs are chilled and firm, remove them from the molds or liners and transfer them to an airtight container for storage.

- Store the vanilla almond butter fat bombs in the refrigerator until ready to enjoy.

COOKING TIPS

- Use unsweetened almond butter for the best texture and flavor in the fat bombs. You can also use other nut butters such as cashew butter or peanut butter if preferred.
- If you prefer a sweeter fat bomb, you can add more powdered erythritol or sweetener of choice to the mixture. To get the right sweetness level, taste as you proceed.
- For added crunch and flavor, you can mix chopped nuts such as almonds, pecans, or walnuts into the fat bomb mixture before chilling.
- If you don't have silicone molds or mini muffin liners, you can also pour the mixture into an ice cube tray to create individual fat bombs.

HEALTH BENEFITS

- Almond butter is a nutritious source of healthy fats, protein, and fiber, which help keep you feeling full and satisfied. It also offers vital nutrients like potassium, magnesium, and vitamin E.
- Coconut oil is rich in medium-chain triglycerides (MCTs), a type of fat that is easily absorbed and converted into energy by the body. MCTs have been linked to various health benefits, including improved metabolism, weight management, and cognitive function.
- Erythritol is a sugar alcohol that provides sweetness without the calories or blood sugar spike associated with regular sugar. It is also tooth-friendly and does not promote tooth decay.

NUTRITIONAL VALUES (PER SERVING, BASED ON 1 FAT BOMB):

- **Calories**: 120
- **Total Fat**: 11g
- **Saturated Fat**: 6g
- **Cholesterol**: 0mg
- **Sodium**: 10mg
- **Total Carbohydrates**: 4g
- **Dietary Fiber**: 2g
- **Sugars**: 1g
- **Protein**: 3g

NOTE: Nutritional values may vary depending on the specific brands and quantities of ingredients used. Adjustments can be made to the recipe to suit individual dietary preferences and requirements.

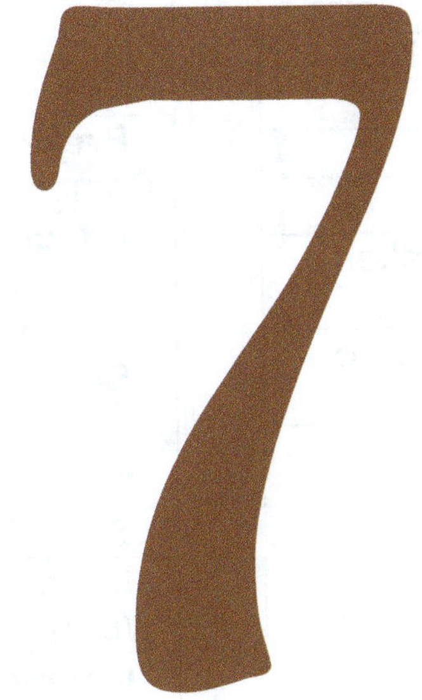

7

BONUS

DR. LESLIE J. STEEN

14-DAYS MEAL PLAN

DAY 1

- **Breakfast**: Spinach and Feta Omelette
- **Lunch**: Tuna Salad Stuffed Bell Peppers
- **Dinner**: Grilled Chicken Caesar Salad
- **Snack**: Cheese and Pepperoni Roll-Ups

DAY 2

- **Breakfast**: Coconut Flour Pancakes with Sugar-Free Syrup
- **Lunch**: Zucchini Noodles with Pesto and Cherry Tomatoes
- **Dinner**: Baked Lemon Herb Salmon
- **Snack**: Guacamole with Low-Carb Veggie Sticks

DAY 3

- **Breakfast**: Avocado and Bacon Breakfast Bowl
- **Lunch**: Turkey and Avocado Lettuce Wraps
- **Dinner**: Cauliflower Crust Pizza with Pepperoni and Mushrooms
- **Snack**: Spicy Buffalo Cauliflower Bites

DAY 4

- **Breakfast**: Classic Bacon and Eggs
- Lunch: Keto-Friendly Broccoli Cheddar Soup
- **Dinner**: Spicy Shrimp Stir-Fry with Cauliflower Rice
- **Snack**:* Almond Flour Crackers with Cream Cheese and Smoked Salmon

DAY 5

- **Breakfast**: Berries and Cream Parfait
- **Lunch**: Tuna Salad Stuffed Bell Peppers
- **Dinner**: Garlic Butter Steak Bites
- **Snack**: Lemon Coconut Fat Bombs

DAY 6

- **Breakfast**: Peanut Butter Chocolate **Chip Cookies (Sugar-Free)**
- **Lunch**: Grilled Portobello Mushroom Burger with Avocado
- **Dinner**: Baked Lemon Herb Salmon
- **Snack**: Spicy Buffalo Cauliflower Bites

DAY 7

- **Breakfast**: Vanilla Almond Butter Fat Bombs
- **Lunch**: Keto-Friendly Coleslaw with Homemade Dressing
- **Dinner**: Grilled Chicken Caesar Salad
- **Snack**: Cucumber Avocado Salsa

DAY 8

- **Breakfast**: Spinach and Feta Omelette
- **Lunch**: Turkey and Avocado Lettuce Wraps
- **Dinner**: Garlic Parmesan Roasted Brussels Sprouts
- **Snack** Cheese and Pepperoni Roll-Ups

DAY 9

- **Breakfast**: Avocado and Bacon Breakfast Bowl
- **Lunch**: Zucchini Noodles with Pesto and Cherry Tomatoes
- **Dinner**: Spicy Shrimp Stir-Fry with Cauliflower Rice
- **Snack**: Guacamole with Low-Carb Veggie Sticks

DAY 10

Breakfast: Coconut Flour Pancakes with Sugar-Free Syrup
- **Lunch**: Tuna Salad Stuffed Bell Peppers
- **Dinner**: Cauliflower Crust Pizza with Pepperoni and Mushrooms
- **Snack**: Almond Flour Crackers with Cream Cheese and Smoked Salmon

DAY 11

- **Breakfast**: Classic Bacon and Eggs
- **Lunch**: Keto-Friendly Broccoli Cheddar Soup
- **Dinner**: Grilled Portobello Mushroom Burger with Avocado
- **Snack**: Lemon Coconut Fat Bombs

DAY 12

- **Breakfast**: Berries and Cream Parfait
- **Lunch**: Turkey and Avocado Lettuce Wraps
- **Dinner**: Garlic Butter Steak Bites
- **Snack**: Spicy Buffalo Cauliflower Bites

DAY 13

- **Breakfast**: Peanut Butter Chocolate

Chip Cookies (Sugar-Free)
- **Lunch**: Keto-Friendly Coleslaw with Homemade Dressing
- **Dinner**: Baked Lemon Herb Salmon
- **Snack**: Cucumber Avocado Salsa

DAY 14:

- **Breakfast**: Vanilla Almond Butter Fat Bombs
- **Lunch**: Spinach and Feta Omelette
- **Dinner**: Grilled Chicken Caesar Salad
- **Snack**: Cheese and Pepperoni Roll-Ups

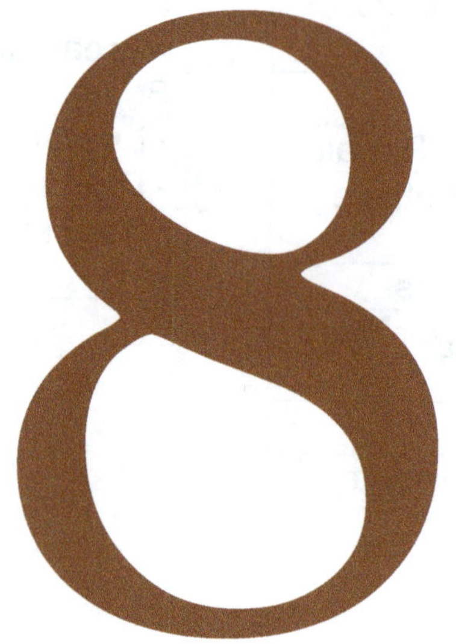

CONCLUSION

DR. LESLIE J. STEEN

Congratulations on completing your journey through the "Atkins Diet Cookbook 2024"! We hope this culinary adventure has provided you with a wealth of delicious and nutritious recipes to support your Atkins lifestyle.

In this cookbook, we've explored a wide variety of recipes ranging from satisfying breakfast options to mouthwatering desserts, all carefully crafted to align with the principles of the Atkins diet. Whether you're looking to kickstart your day with a protein-packed breakfast, enjoy a satisfying lunch, or indulge in a guilt-free dessert, you'll find something to suit your tastes and dietary needs within these pages.

Throughout this cookbook, we've emphasized the importance of choosing wholesome, nutrient-dense ingredients and incorporating a balance of protein, healthy fats, and fiber-rich carbohydrates into your meals. By focusing on whole foods and minimizing processed ingredients, you can nourish your body while enjoying flavorful and satisfying meals.

We've also provided cooking tips, health benefits, and nutritional information for each recipe to help you make informed choices about your food and understand how it fits into your overall dietary goals. Whether you're aiming to lose weight, maintain a healthy lifestyle, or manage a specific health condition, the Atkins diet can be a valuable tool to support your journey to better health and well-being.

As you continue on your Atkins journey, remember that success is not just about what you eat, but also how you approach your lifestyle overall. Incorporating regular physical activity, staying hydrated, getting enough sleep, and managing stress are all important factors that contribute to your overall health and well-being.

We hope this cookbook has inspired you to get creative in the kitchen, explore new flavors and ingredients, and discover the joy of nourishing your body with delicious, wholesome foods. Remember to listen to your body, honor your hunger and fullness cues, and make choices that support your long-term health and happiness.

We appreciate you coming along for this culinary journey. Here's to your health, happiness, and many more delicious meals to come!

Happy cooking!

DR. LESLIE J. STEEN

REVIEW

Dear Readers,

As you close the pages of the "Atkins Diet Cookbook 2024," we hope you've found inspiration, delicious recipes, and valuable insights to support your journey toward a healthier lifestyle. Your feedback is incredibly important to us, and we would be grateful if you could take a moment to share your thoughts by leaving a review.

Your review will not only help other readers decide if this cookbook is right for them but also provide us with valuable insights into what you enjoyed and how we can continue to improve. Whether you loved trying out the recipes, found the cooking tips helpful, or have suggestions for future editions, your feedback is invaluable to us.

Leaving a review is quick and easy. Simply visit the website or platform where you purchased or accessed the cookbook, navigate to the book's page, and look for the option to leave a review. You can share your thoughts on the recipes, the organization of the cookbook, the clarity of the instructions, or any other aspect that resonated with you.

If you're unsure what to include in your review, here are a few questions to consider:
- Which recipes did you enjoy the most, and why?
- Were the cooking tips helpful in preparing the recipes?
- Did you find the nutritional information provided useful?
- How would you rate the overall organization and layout of the cookbook?
- Would you recommend this cookbook to others who are interested in following the Atkins diet?

Your honest feedback will not only help us continue to improve but also assist fellow readers in making informed decisions about whether this cookbook is the right fit for them.

Thank you for taking the time to share your thoughts. We truly appreciate your support and look forward to hearing from you!

Warm regards,

DR. LESLIE J. STEEN